The Girl Who Cried Brave

A Story of Strength and Courage

SARAH TOMLIN

Published by
Fideli Publishing, Inc.
119 W. Morgan St.
Martinsville, IN 46151

www.FideliPublishing.com

*Hard times forge a
strong and courageous soul.*

Table of Contents

CHAPTER 1

The Pit

"In my distress I called to the Lord, and he answered me. From deep in the realm of the dead I called for help, and you listened to my cry."

—Jonah 2:2, NIV

I was in a deep, dark pit. Dirt caked beneath my fingernails. My muscles screamed. Every limb trembled with exhaustion, but I clawed at the crumbling walls, refusing to surrender. I reached again—fingers aching, heart pounding, breath ragged. I scraped and dragged myself upward, inch by grueling inch, forcing motion into limbs that begged to give up.

The wall fought back, gravity pressed down, but I pushed harder.

Finally, near collapse, I hooked an elbow over the edge. My chest cleared the rim. I sprawled forward, cheek pressed against the cool ground, gasping, barely stable. I didn't fall back in. Not this time. I made it—today.

But could I survive the climb again tomorrow? The task felt Sisyphean: both effortful and exhausting.

That pit mirrored my depression. Every morning, I woke again at the bottom—cold, heavy, suffocating. I didn't just feel low; I felt buried alive. Climbing out required every shred of willpower I had, and even then, I questioned why I bothered. Death didn't scare me—*wanting* it did. The pull toward the end whispered louder each day. I hadn't made a plan yet, but the idea coiled around me, tightening.

By this time in my life, I had drifted far from God. I honestly hadn't given Him much thought. I grew up a "Christian" but had never encountered God. I grew up in church, I had just drifted away. As a kid, our family's church was our second home. We went every Sunday (except during the summers, when my parents took a break from everything) for service, every Monday for bell choir practice, every Wednesday for singing choir practice, and occasionally an extra day was thrown in there for a special occasion. We were fifty minutes away from church, each way. It was my brother, sister, and I, and our friends the Johnsons, who had four children. The seven of us played endlessly in that church in Ithaca, New York. It was our kingdom and we were royalty there.

We knew where every corner, every closet, every nook and cranny, every hidey hole and passageway was. We knew where the spare props for plays were kept, which doors were locked and which weren't, and we knew the industrial kitchen inside and out with its stainless-steel counters and sink. We even got to play with the organ once in a great while. This had to be done under parental supervision and only when it was off. But it was still fascinating. I would flick the switches up and down, press down the floor pedals, pull knobs, push buttons, and hit the keys, pretending I could create a beautiful symphony of sound.

If I close my eyes even now I can still picture the soft crimson carpet upstairs, the medium brown tile flecked with green downstairs. I can recall the difference in smell between them. Upstairs had a softer smell—it smelled of the somewhat-new carpet, a faint lingering coffee smell, and a slight hint of the wood trim around. Downstairs was like almost every church basement across America. Not a dank and moldy smell, no, but concrete and cinder blocks. We spent our entire childhood coming up with games, playing tag in the parking lot, laughing on the playground, and occasionally playing hide-and-seek in the dark but more often inside the church. We knew exactly how loud we could be to prevent incurring the wrath of our parents. Too much noise and they would be able to hear us in between songs. The older kids (Chloe Johnson, my sister Maureen, and later on my brother James) would shush the younger ones when our shouting was verging on bringing a parent out who would definitely put us in our place. No good would come of aggravating the adults, so we learned to police ourselves.

Having spent so much time in church, you'd think I would have grown up a strong Christian, walking closely with the Lord. Honestly, I'm not sure why I didn't. That's just not how it unfolded. I didn't realize it at the time, but I had made myself my own god. I did what I wanted, when I wanted, with little regard for anything else. I only cared about myself. My needs and desires took center stage in the play of my life. I'm ashamed to admit it now, but it's the truth. I wish I had recognized it sooner.

I struggled with bouts of depression starting in my teens. Each time, I would pull out of it after a few months. But having kids changed everything. With two little ones demanding every second of my attention, I started to drown. It felt like treading water with weights tied to my ankles. Keeping my head above water drained every bit of energy year after year. Eventually, I no longer had the strength to stay afloat. I gave in to the pull and began sinking.

On what may have been the darkest day, my husband had just left with our kids to take them to daycare and then drive on to work. For no reason I could understand, tears suddenly flooded out. The sobs came in waves, relentless, as they carved a small, warm river down my face. I felt broken—like a dam had burst open inside me.

It was from that dark place that I cried out to God for help. Again and again, I pleaded, "Please, bring me home. I just want to go home." What I meant was clear—I was ready to leave this life behind. I wanted to be in Heaven. I was done. I was ready to die.

I wish I could tell you there was a miraculous moment—an overwhelming rush of the Holy Spirit that instantly made every-thing better. But it didn't happen like that. There was no dramatic shift. It was slow, almost unnoticeable at first. I don't know why

God chose to help me. He didn't have to. I hadn't given Him the time of day; why would He give me His? And yet, He did. Little by little, He met me in the darkness. It was a new feeling—one I didn't recognize at first.

It started with small coincidences—the kind that don't feel like coincidences at all in hindsight. The first came when a co-worker casually suggested I try a Christian music station. I figured it couldn't hurt, so I gave it a shot. Around that time, "God Only Knows" by For King and Country had just been released. It played multiple times a day while I worked, and every time it came on, it felt like God was speaking straight to me. Even now, when I hear that song, I feel the tears rise and sense God gently reminding me that He's still here. The Bible says, "Draw near to God, and He will draw near to you." "Seek, and you shall find." But that first step? It's ours to take. God is always there—patient, steady, waiting.

That online Christian station aired two hours of preaching every day—four pastors, each delivering a half-hour message grounded in Scripture. I started tuning in regularly and even began reading a few Bible verses on my own. At the time, I had no idea how to read the Bible. It felt confusing and overwhelming. I didn't understand how the Old and New Testaments connected—or if they even did. But I was trying. Each night, I'd read a verse, and then—like clockwork—a pastor would preach on that exact verse the very next day. The first time, I chalked it up to coincidence. But it kept happening. Week after week. It was starting to feel a little... uncanny. Small coincidences.

Eventually, I started trying to make sense of it. *Maybe I'm just reading the Bible in the same order the pastors are preaching,* I thought. *That would explain it.* So, I decided to test it. I flipped to a completely different part of the Bible—Psalm 99. The words hit me hard: "*They called to the Lord, and He answered them... O Lord our God, You answered Your people.*" In that moment, I felt the presence of God so clearly, as if He were telling me directly, *I hear you. I'm answering your prayer.* And then—just like before—the very next day, a preacher quoted that exact verse.

By this point, I was convinced—these weren't just coincidences. This had been happening nearly every day for over two weeks. God was reaching out to me, gently, tenderly. And I could feel it. The more I filled myself with Him, and the more of myself I poured out, the clearer my mind became. The crushing weight of depression began to lift, not all at once, but gradually—like the morning sun dissolving the fog. It was slow, but it was real.

I want to say that I understand depression is multifaceted and that just wanting to get better is not enough, and solely praying will not be enough for everyone. Some people have deep trauma, fear, or anxiety that will need counseling to work through. I recognized at the time that I needed to attack my depression from multiple angles, so I was also making sure to exercise, spend time in nature, take certain vitamins, get good sleep, and limit how much alcohol I was drinking. Since then, I've also learned cold showers help (as cold as you can for as long as you can take it). There is science behind this and research backs it up. Is it fun? Absolutely not. But is it effective? You bet. Trust me on the cold shower! Those are the things that seem to help me to this day. But the single most important thing is focusing on God daily. When I prioritize Him, everything else seems to fall into place and my mood lifts.

I still struggle with the beast that is depression from time to time. In fact, it would come back later in my journey, trying once again to consume me. The enemy knows our weaknesses—he remembers what worked before to pull us away from God, and he's not afraid to try the same tactics again. But now, I know the truth: my joy isn't rooted in my circumstances. It's deeper than that. *Joy comes in the morning* (Psalm 30:5), and each new day is another chance to rise, to reset, to choose hope. My forever joy rests in knowing that Jesus has already done the hard work— once and for all.

This drawing closer between God and I culminated in a beautiful moment one night. I was driving home from a massage (an indulgence I allow myself every once in awhile) and a light-ning storm lit up the sky. It was one of those perfect, warm spring nights when jackets are no longer needed—the first taste of sum-mer lingering just ahead. The air buzzed with a mix of excite-ment and quiet expectation, scented with freshly cut grass and blooming flowers. The air felt electric. You could *smell* the sea-sons changing. The storm stayed far in the distance—no thunder, no rain—just streaks of lightning dancing across the sky from one horizon to the other. It was absolutely breathtaking.

The drive home was very short; there was only enough time for one song. In that space, the song "Light Up the Sky" by The

Afters came on. My car filled with the song about God lighting up the sky. Once again, I felt God speaking to my soul through the circumstances around me. It was an amazing experience. Only if you have ever felt like you were truly in the presence of the living God will you understand the awe and wonder I felt in that moment. It was when I knew God was with me, and He was for me.

Negative emotions and behaviors can be tricky in that they often travel together. The dominant emotion may not be the true source of a problem, but it can hold our attention and focus while the real problem maker is silently lurking in the background. Emotions like anger and anxiety go hand in hand with alcohol, outbursts, depression, and so on. When my children were little, I definitely struggled with some anger that had its roots in depression. God did not want me to stay in this anger and He cared too much to leave me the way I was. He isn't always a whisper. Sometimes, as I found out, He is the opposite.

My daughter Grace was three at the time and a handful. n those early years, she was incredibly headstrong and, frankly, pretty mean. A classic "bossy girl," as some might say. We clashed constantly. I remember nights of yelling at the top of my lungs, slamming her bedroom door shut, then stomping up the stairs in pure frustration. One night, completely exasperated, I turned to Bill and declared, "I can't live with her for fifteen more years— she's going to boarding school." And I meant it. I actually got online and started looking. That is, until I saw the tuition. One glance at that price tag, and I quickly changed my mind. Side note: don't worry, Grace is a lovely child now. But at the time, I had my doubts it would turn around.

On the night that God figuratively swatted the back of my head, I was dealing with Grace's obstinate attitude yet again and things were escalating. I was so angry at Grace that I couldn't see straight. I grabbed her tiny arm and yanked. If it hurt her, she did not let on but in retrospect it was way too hard. God's voice this time was not a whisper, it was loud and stern: "She's my daughter too!"

It was like touching a red-hot stove. Stunned, I pulled back. In that moment, I took stock of where I was and how I had gotten there—so much anger, all of it pent up and poured out on this little person who didn't deserve it. God was stepping in, claiming her as His own and making it clear that I was not to mistreat her. He was showing me that this path of unchecked anger, it was dangerous. It was leading me somewhere I didn't want to go, somewhere I might not be able to pull back from. And He did not approve. *"For the Lord disciplines the one He loves,"* Hebrews 12:6 says. That night, I felt that discipline. And I knew I had earned it.

God was breaking up the hard ground in my life. Like a barren field, He tilled it all. Got rid of weeds. Cultivated. Planted. He was working the soil of my heart so that the roots could grow deep and strong. Pruning the vines to produce fruit later. He did not answer my prayers to come home and He still hasn't. But He doesn't always answer our prayers the way we want Him to. The purpose of prayer isn't to get everything you ask for. It's not a transaction—it's a relationship. Sometimes, the things we go through are meant to grow us, to shape us into who we're meant to be.

The relationship with God a lot like parenting. Sometimes, God says "no," just like you have to tell your children no. When you tell your child it's time for bed, even though they beg to stay up, it doesn't mean you don't love them. In fact, it's because you love them that you say no. It's the same with God; except He sees the future. For those who serve Him, there is a distinct purpose, one that was set in motion before time began (see Ephesians 1:4, Hebrews 13:21, and Romans 8:28). And everything He allows is part of fulfilling that purpose. Sometimes, and these are the hardest times, He will allow bad things to happen to us because it is an opportunity for us to grow. I would find out more about this later.

CHAPTER 2

A Whisper from Within

"For God does speak—now one way, now another—though no one perceives it. In a dream, in a vision of the night, when deep sleep falls on people as they slumber in their beds, he may speak in their ears and terrify them with warnings, to turn them from wrongdoing and keep them from pride, to preserve them from the pit, their lives from perishing by the sword."

—Job 33:14-18 NIV

It was at this time when I was climbing out of my depression that God first reached out to me in my dreams. Or rather, what I call a dream, though it wasn't really one. It happened in that strange, in-between space as I was waking up—half-asleep, half-aware, eyes still closed. Semiconscious. I can't prove it. I can't fully explain it. And whenever I try, I stumble over the words. But I *know* what I heard. I felt it in my soul. It was a whisper. Not something born in my own mind, but something other.

It made my eyes snap open. It was as clear and close as if my husband had leaned in and whispered in my ear… except it came from within. It whispered, "Joshua, 1, 8, 9."

Now fully awake, I lay there, perplexed. Somehow, deep down, my soul *knew*—it was the One who made me, whispering in that moment. The Creator. But… *was Joshua even a book in the Bible?* I had always owned a Bible, but rarely—if ever—used it. I wasn't even sure where to begin. I reached for the Bible I had recently placed beside my bed and started flipping through the books. I didn't know if Joshua was in the New Testament or the Old. I wasn't even sure I *wanted* it to be there. What would it mean if it was? Was Joshua just a name? A character? Or an actual book?

Dreams are usually just silly, fragmented bits of reality. But this had felt different than any dream. I scanned the table of contents nervously, heart beating faster. The idea that this could be something real—something *divine*—left me unsettled in a way I couldn't explain.

And then, there it was. I found it. It turns out that Joshua is a book in the Bible as well as a character in it. Joshua was a mighty warrior and took charge, as decreed by God, right after Moses and the Exodus from Egypt. I read Joshua 1:8–9 that day to see what God had to say to me. It reads, "Keep this book of the Law always on your lips; meditate on it day and night, so that you may be careful to do everything written in it. Then you will be prosperous and successful. Have I not commanded you? Be strong and courageous. Do not be afraid; do not be discouraged, for the Lord your God will be with you wherever you go." (NIV)

I sat there and stared silently. Once again God was telling me that He was with me. I was amazed at what God said to me through His Word that day. He was with me! I had a few other dreams from God over the next couple years. Whenever I felt His presence in those dreams, believe me, it was the most beautiful feeling I have ever known. I could feel His presence in a special way. I will forever crave more of it. It was a peace so deep, a wholeness and rightness so complete, it overwhelmed me. It made me want to change my entire life just to feel more of it. That longing stirred something in me, and my appetite to know more about God became insatiable. I couldn't get enough.

I ended up joining a small group through my church, hungry to learn, to grow, to draw closer. We read and discussed the book *30 Days to Understanding the Bible* by Max Anders. It explains the Bible in terms of the types of books, the time period they were written, the general stories in each book, and how each book is relevant to the overarching story. The book and our discussions in the group began to unlock something. I felt like I had been given a key to a secret room full of ancient knowledge. Now that I could finally begin to understand the Bible, it suddenly leapt off the pages as if alive; it was no longer relegated to boring sermons that had no relevance to today's world.

I downloaded a Bible app so I could read the Bible daily and do devotionals. I listened to *The Bible Recap* podcast by Tara-Leigh Cobble and watched *The Bible Project* videos on YouTube.

Each time I connected with God's word I understood more and more of the Bible. Before it had been a rather dull, even boring, account of some incongruent stories and a long list of names. Now it was one story, a rich tapestry woven full of metaphors that still apply to this day, despite being four thousand years old.

Over the next several years, my relationship with the Lord blossomed and matured. Like any relationship, it didn't happen overnight. It took time, intention, and a lot of grace. But slowly, steadily, things began to change. The world, once a place of tumult where East felt like West and up felt like down, started to make sense. When grounded in Jesus, everything found its place. Scripture says to guard your heart and to meditate on Heaven (see Proverbs 4:23 and Colossians 3:2). I began to examine myself deeper than I ever had. What was I putting in my head? What was I choosing daily, either subconsciously or otherwise? I began to guard my heart and to turn my thoughts more often to Heaven. I paid more attention to what I was watching and listening to. These small steps added up to a more positive impact on my mental health.

God began prompting me to cut the callus off my heart—to love others more deeply, to pursue justice with compassion, to care for the downtrodden, and to give more freely to the causes that matter to Him. He was softening me, reshaping me. But it wasn't until I truly understood the weight of sin (how serious it is) that I could begin to grasp just how desperately I needed God.

I know sin isn't exactly a fun topic. But it's fundamental to having a real relationship with God. We tend to think we're doing pretty well with sin. Even when we look at the Ten Commandments in plain English. I mean, I don't have idols or other gods. I haven't murdered anyone. I've checked the boxes, right? That's what I used to think. But it wasn't until I started listening to people who truly understood the depth of Scripture, experts who unpacked the Hebrew roots and God's intent behind each commandment, that I realized how much more they mean. An idol isn't just a statue. It's anything we praise or give more attention to than God. Murder can be as simple as tearing someone down with our words. Every commandment speaks to the condition of the human heart, which, if we're honest, is easily led astray. God has always known this. He knew it from the very beginning. It just took me my whole life to see it.

Realizing how many things God actually considers sinful suddenly made one thing clear: getting through life without sinning is *impossible*. God looked through all time and also knew this would be the case. That's the whole reason He created a way to reconcile us to Himself through the sacrifice of Jesus. And as if that weren't enough, He continues to draw near. He saves us not just once, but every single day. He saved *me* from crushing depression. Through that, I learned how to lean on Him. I learned what I believe. It's a good thing I did, because I'm not sure I would have made it through what was to come next if I hadn't.

CHAPTER 3

Mysterious Symptoms

"So do not fear, for I am with you; do not be dismayed, for I am your God. I will strengthen you and help you; I will uphold you with my righteous right hand."

—Isaiah 41:10 NIV

My little dog Toby wanted to go outside. I sighed, finished my case on the computer for work, pushed out my chair, and stood up. *Uh oh.* Something was wrong. I couldn't quite put my finger on it, but something felt ... off. I took a step with my right leg. That seemed normal enough. But when I tried to take a step with my left leg, it was as if the signal from my brain halted at my hip and then traveled through sludge the rest of the way. It was like my leg was saying, "You want me to do *what* now? Sorry, can't quite make that out. The line's full of static."

I half dragged my leg slowly forward to where I wanted it. I tried again. Right leg—normal. Left leg—drag and delay. *What is going on?* I tried not to panic. My knee felt like jelly. I had a hard time supporting my weight; the knee kept buckling. The thigh muscles in that leg felt like I had done squats to the point of muscle failure. I precariously took step after step, slowly advancing toward the stairs.

Am I going to need a walker before I'm forty? The thought hit me hard. *This must be multiple sclerosis.* I had been suspecting it for weeks. The strange, creeping symptoms had started in April 2021. One spring afternoon, as I walked up the big hill toward my house, I felt my left toes catch and drag on the pavement—just a couple times, but enough to notice. Back at home, I sank into my trusty recliner and stared at my feet. *What is wrong with you?* I wondered, as if they might answer me. My left leg felt off—weak somehow. That's when I noticed it: my right foot was pointed straight up toward the ceiling, while my left hung limp, slouched toward the floor. I tried to flex, to bring both feet up toward my knees. The right one responded immediately. The left? Only made it halfway. *This isn't good,* I thought.

After that first incident, my body started doing things I couldn't explain. Strange, unpredictable things it had never done before. I felt like a marionette, as if someone else were pulling the strings, and I could never quite tell what movement was coming next. My hands would curl up uncontrollably, twisting into distorted shapes that reminded me of an old witch's claws. If I gripped something heavy, my hand would lock in place. I couldn't open it using the muscles in that arm—I had to pry the object free with my other hand, then physically straighten out my fingers.

My legs and abdominal muscles twitched constantly, as though electricity was buzzing just beneath the surface. At night, my legs jerked and kicked involuntarily, waking me from sleep again and again. Sometimes it felt like a bug was crawling across my skin. My eyes would lose focus, and when I strained to see clearly, they darted back and forth uncontrollably. But the hardest part of all was the weakness. My muscles just didn't have the strength they once did.

I've mostly been pretty fit my whole life. In high school, I played soccer, basketball, and softball. In college, I even had a brief stint on the rowing team. Starting in junior high, I rode horses and did some competitive jumping in the arena. Before I got pregnant with my son, I was doing sprint-distance triathlons. (Full disclosure: I can also rock a nap like nobody's business, and doing nothing is still one of my favorite pastimes.)

But overall, I've always been fairly athletic. I tend to cycle through phases of being "in shape" and "out of shape," and just before everything started going sideways, I was in a motivated stretch—running, lifting weights, and seeing enough progress to feel good about it. Then, all of a sudden, I was struggling just to brush my daughter's hair. My arm felt like it was full of lead. My shoulders ached, and they felt as exhausted as if I'd been lifting weights all morning. I had to pause and take breaks between strokes with the brush. Something wasn't right.

My regular doctor offered a brain MRI to me when I went to see her about these neurological symptoms. She gave me a referral to a neurologist, but I hadn't been able to get in to see him.

Because of Covid and shortages in the specialty, the neurologist she referred me to had a three-month wait list. I made the appointment for July. I failed to see what else I could do. No one was treating this like it was an emergency. But to me, it *felt* like one. *I can't wait that long*, I thought, but knew I would have to. Still, my symptoms were so alarming to me that I was worried. In the meantime, all sorts of scenarios and rare disorders ran through my mind. All the while, I had to keep going, had to keep dealing with the spasms, the constant twitches, and the debilitating weakness that made even the simplest tasks feel monumental.

Toby's soft whimper drew my mind back to the present task of getting to the door. *Well, at least my leg is still complying, even though the message is delayed and the going is slow,* I thought. A new obstacle now loomed before me: the stairs. I was not sure if I would be able to lift my leg enough to ascend. The chore was normally thoughtless. I stood with my toes a few inches from the step and prepared myself. *If my leg won't lift by itself, I will have to use my arms to lift it.* Here we go. ...

I focused solely on getting my leg up that step. I thought if I could just concentrate hard enough it would make up for my muscles not doing their job. The leg ever-so-slowly rose, rose, inch by inch. It was so slow! *Come on!* I was ready to give up, thinking that this just wouldn't happen. *Should I call 911? No, what would they even do? What would I tell them? "Hello, yes I feel weird. Can you let my dog out?"* I nearly laughed at the thought.

Finally, I got my foot clear of the lip of the step. I planted it firmly. *Uh-oh, now will it be able to hold me while I put all my weight on it to get the other leg up? Why didn't I just start with my right leg?*

If only the thought had occurred to me before attempting these stairs! I shifted my weight and slowly added more and more weight to the left leg until I felt confident it would hold. I brought the right leg up with ease. The signals to that leg were functioning normally so it was fast. Now I again used the right to begin the climb, then got the left to follow suit. Progress was agonizingly slow.

Toby grew more and more impatient. He danced from one front leg to the other, fervently glancing from me to the door. He scratched at the door. Then he snorted, which was his way of showing he was annoyed. Internally I laughed because I couldn't blame him, and he was so stinking cute. Most of us are so used to instant gratification in this world that waiting has become nearly obsolete. Anything that hinders us is irritating at once.

I hear you; I'm coming ... eventually.

I did make it up those stairs—it just took a lot longer than I wanted it to. I ran out of patience a couple of times. But I made it. After about five or ten minutes, which felt more like half an hour, my leg finally started to feel normal again. I was growing increasingly frustrated with these bizarre episodes. *How am I supposed to explain this to a neurologist,* I wondered, *when the episodes only last a few minutes?* How do you describe something that disappears before you can even put it into words?

It would've been easy for a doctor to dismiss my symptoms since they lasted only seconds at times. But those seconds were deeply disruptive to my life. I type for a living. And typing with weak arms, while my muscles contracted all day long, made work incredibly difficult. Keeping my hands from curling into fists became a constant, exhausting effort. It felt like rubber bands were wrapped tight around my fingers, and just holding them in a natural, open position took focus and the strength of my forearms. By the end of each day, my arms were worn out from trying to meet my productivity quota. Still, I trudged on. What else was I to do?

I didn't think it was that serious until I saw my doctor and she said, "I can fill out FMLA paperwork if you bring it in. Many people with something like this can't finish a workday and need an alternate schedule."

That hit me like a sucker punch.

I wasn't expecting it. As a healthy person in my thirties, I had never imagined needing help just to do my job. And it's not like my work was physically demanding—I sat in front of a computer reviewing medical claims all day, for crying out loud! But now, not having full control of my own body? That was uncharted territory. *Will I really need FMLA?* I was scared.

The unknowns were piling up fast. My doctor was ordering a brain MRI. My muscles weren't cooperating. And the fear was creeping in. That moment felt like a turning point. It was a lot to hit me all at once. But the hits? They would keep on coming.

CHAPTER 4

An Unconventional Meeting

I found the one my heart loves.
—Song of Songs 3:4 NIV

I met my husband Bill when I was eighteen. And it was anything but conventional. This was August 2001, a mere month before the terrorist attacks of September 11th that caused a permanent fracture in our country and separated our history into "before" and "after". At the time, I was interested in forensics (a fascination I shared with many others, even before shows like *CSI* hit the airwaves).

Thanks to a connection through my dad, who volunteered for the local sheriff's department's boat patrol, I landed a job for the summer. My parents lived on a large lake that was tough to police with such a small department, so the patrol needed extra help. The role? Mostly public relations. A handful of other eighteen-year-olds and I spent our days cruising the lake, chatting with boaters, and working on our tans. I know—tough gig, right?

That May, a small group of friends in their early twenties threw a beach party and decided to take a boat out on the lake. What they didn't account for was the brutal chill of the water. In the Finger Lakes region of New York, the water stays bone-chillingly cold well into spring—often hovering in the fifties, even when the air warms into the seventies or higher. It's a deadly mix that catches someone off guard every few years. They assume it's safe because the sun is out, but the water tells a different story.

Sometimes alcohol is involved in the decision to jump in, sometimes it's just poor judgment. But when you hit water that cold, your body only has minutes to survive. Tragically, that's exactly what happened to a young man that spring. He didn't make it out.

The young man's family was desperate to recover his body. Two search teams had already tried and failed. That's when the Trident Foundation was called in for another attempt. This was no longer a search—it was a mission to bring a grieving family some peace.

Bill had first seen the Trident Foundation in action during a recovery mission near Fort Benning, Georgia, where he was stationed with the Army at the time. Watching them work left a lasting impression. Most of the crew were retired military—disciplined, capable, and deeply mission-driven. After seeing their professionalism and heart, Bill knew this was an outfit he wanted to spend more time with. So, he signed up to volunteer.

A few months later, he was asked if he wanted to go on a mission in central New York. He was in one of several trucks that rumbled onto the scene where the group of young people had last been seen. Gear was unloaded, equipment checked, and the quiet resolve of the team settled in. The spot was in a beautiful park right on Seneca Lake. These serious-looking men poured out of their vehicles and began unloading this equally serious-looking gear. They were talking and joking, all very familiar with each other. They were not crass but they also weren't formal. They were professional but personable. They were somehow laid-back and jovial but moving with a purpose. It's what I now know is the way confident military and former military service members all fall into a rhythm together right away. A camaraderie.

I thought I noticed the youngest, handsomest guy with the group spot me. He began laying out gear and counting. Bill has since told me that he was just doing this to get closer to me. Later that work day we struck up a conversation. It was instant chemistry between us and we talked with ease for hours. As soon as we started work again the next morning at seven, we found an excuse to be near one another and talked for most of the day again.

I thought we had kept things pretty professional and hoped that would be enough to keep any whispers at bay. It wasn't. Everyone on the site noticed. By the end of the second day, the guy in charge of the group had gotten my phone number from the undersheriff and passed it along to Bill, telling him he needed to call me.

Lucky for me, he did call me. He even asked me out on a date. We spent the next three nights in a row going on dates.

Dates that started after our workday ended, which was around nine at night. We would head out for a bite to eat at ten or eleven, sit on park benches, look at the stars, and talk some more. There may have been a few stellar kisses in there as well. I would creep my car as quietly as possible into my parents' garage at four in the morning, knowing I had only two hours to sleep before getting up again to go back to work. This is part of the gift of youth, because I now need a nap after work if we are even going to watch a movie on the couch after eight.

It was after our first date that I first heard what I perceived as God's voice. I parked my teal 1992 Volkswagen Jetta in the garage and sat there for a moment, giddy from the instant, undeniable connection that we'd had. Then, out of nowhere, I heard a voice echo in my head. It wasn't mine. It came spontaneously, as a thought that was just *given* to me: *You're going to marry him.*

My immediate reaction was to argue with the voice. *That's nonsense, I just met him!* I mean honestly, what on earth would you think? Funny thing about the Lord, though—He means what He says. After those first three dates, Bill had to go back to Georgia. Just two weeks later, he asked if he could fly me down to visit him. We were married a little over two years after that, in the wake of his first deployment and with the shadow of a second one already looming. The first deployment lasted eight brutal months. I finally felt like I had him all to myself again. Just four months after he returned, as we were getting ready to make the thirteen-hour drive to see our families for Christmas, we got gut-punched.

The chain of command passed down the terrible news: Bill had less than two weeks home for Christmas before heading out on his second deployment. My heart was crushed. It felt like we had drawn a strong first hand in a high-stakes game of Black-jack. But, as they say, the house always wins. I couldn't shake the worry that something might happen this time. I knew how dangerous deployments were. It had already felt miraculous that he'd gotten through one unscathed. Would our luck really hold out?

I decided I didn't want to take that chance. I didn't want to risk losing him without being truly bound to him—not just legally, but emotionally, spiritually. Bonded souls. I didn't want to wait and wonder through another deployment. I wanted to be his wife.

Our love was then and still is a bit of a fairy-tale type of love. I have grown into an adult with him. We've weathered many storms together, with his eight deployments among the worst storms. We have moved up and down the East Coast and across parts of the United States together. He is a deeply caring, fiercely protective, loyal, selfless soul, and it was always so easy for me to love him. You'd think being faced with a wife of failing physical health would be a challenge, or might bring out someone's "true colors." Some might be tempted to tuck tail and run. But not this man. He tackled this problem head-on as befitting of an unflinching soldier. At the time, we were so focused on my plight that we never imagined anything could be wrong with him.

Being in the military, Bill was in excellent shape. He had to make a career of being fit. Exercise was part and parcel to his job.

He was forty-four at the time when I began to have these strange neuromuscular symptoms. He was young, with no family history of any medical problems. His many deployments had given him a lot of close calls. These resulted in some lifelong problems like tinnitus, chronic torn rotator cuff, a torn knee meniscus that would flare up and make his knee swell from time to time, a disc in his lower back that would slip out of place now and then, traumatic brain injury, tuberculosis exposure, and burn pit exposure. You expect such a physical job to take its toll as an unfortunate side effect. But we would be blindsided by a deeper problem.

It was a Saturday when the world came crashing down around me. Bill headed out to run some errands in his usual cheerful mood. We kissed goodbye and exchanged I love you's. I had no idea the day would end with him in the hospital.

I was surprised to have him call me about an hour after he'd left. I answered expecting him to have a mundane question. Perhaps he would ask about whether he should pick something up while he was out or whether the kids already had something he thought he'd buy them. Instead, he said he felt dizzy. He'd been standing in line at the store and had started to feel short of breath. Thinking he just needed air, he had stepped out into the parking lot. Rather than asking if we had enough milk at home, he was asking what I thought he should do with feeling faint and dizzy.

"Maybe you should call an ambulance," I offered.

I'm not going to say that Bill doesn't often take my medical advice. But his next response was that he might try walking around to see if the feeling would fade, and then he might try to drive home if he didn't feel better.

"Do you think you should be driving if you feel like you might faint?" I asked.

He was confident he could do it. A true Army Ranger, through and through. I hung up the phone worried, but if anyone could push his body to the limit, it was my husband. About fifteen minutes later, though, my phone started lighting up—one worrisome text after another.

Feeling worse, going to try to make it home.

Had to stop and pull over.

Called an ambulance, passing out.

I desperately tried calling him. There was no answer. I next tried texting back to get more information. I asked where his location was, what hospital he was going to, was he still conscious, had the ambulance arrived ... all were met with eerie silence. I could feel panic rising in my chest. I didn't know if he was passed out on the side of the road or if he was being helped. And with no known medical conditions, I had no idea what was going on with him. I didn't even know where he was.

I said a quick prayer and tried not to lose it. *Lord, please protect my husband and help him.* With tears stinging my eyes, I tried to reason with myself. If an ambulance had reached him, it would take at least forty-five minutes to an hour for them to assess and either release him or transport him to a hospital. He was likely either with the EMTs or already en route to be admitted. Either way, I would need to sit tight and wait. I wanted to scream, to cry, to do something—anything—but I knew that wouldn't help me find my husband.

I clutched my phone and paced our front lawn for the better part of that hour. No calls. No texts. I was beginning to feel distress. *Time to start calling hospitals.* I tried the first one, connected to the central line, and asked for the Emergency department. When someone in the ER picked up, I said, "I'm looking for my husband who was brought in by ambulance." I gave the woman his name and waited anxiously while she checked the patients. No, he wasn't there.

Ok, try the next one. This time, it was a success (luckily our town is not that big)! I quickly asked the nurse for an update. After a brief hold, she told me they had given him fluids and he was stable. They were waiting on tests. *Hmm.* I was hoping to hear more about what the heck was happening to him, but I was definitely relieved that I had found him and to know he had arrived and was in their care.

Another hour passed before I started getting texts again from Bill. He updated me as best he could while in pain and being worked on. He said the paramedics needed to pull him out of his truck. His blood pressure in the ambulance had been 220/110. He didn't remember much of the ride to the hospital. They were going to take him for a chest CT (a type of scan). They would also run an EKG. His chest was heavy and it felt like there was an elephant sitting on it.

When I was in nursing school, they told us that people having a heart attack often say the exact words: *"It feels like there's an elephant on my chest."* I never forgot that. And now, here was my healthy, forty-four-year-old husband possibly living that moment. How could this be happening?

The next two days while he was in the hospital dragged on like weeks. So many questions, so few answers. And when I did manage to speak briefly with his doctors, trying to get clear information about what was actually going on felt like pulling teeth.

They told me he was having a cardiac event. *Well no kidding!* "What does his EKG look like?" I asked when I got the chance. Even trying to get that little bit of information was difficult. I was texting and calling so many people. So many things to coordinate; to try and string together.

There was also the ordeal of his truck, which had been left in a bank parking lot and needed to be picked up. Having moved to the area just a year prior, I didn't have many people I could rely on to help pick up the slack. Thankfully, the military has a built-in family support group for just such emergencies.

In the Army, this group is called the Family Readiness Group, or FRG for short. Moving is the nature of military life. I don't think I've ever met a military wife who truly 'knew what she was getting into' when she married her serviceman—though civilians often say that to us, as if we were clairvoyants at eighteen or whatever young age we were when we made that decision. Because clearly, we were all making well-informed, carefully weighed life choices back then, right?

An average Army family moves every two years. To say this is hard on the family is an understatement. Finding new doctors, enrolling in new schools, moving boxes, packing tape, PCS (permanent change of station) orders ... these mark the cadence of military family life with the same regularity as the changing of seasons. Fall, winter, spring, summer, move, and repeat for up to twenty years.

In the military, you're rarely, if ever, stationed near your extended family. Moving so often prevents you from getting to know neighbors or having friends for very long. And your actual family can live three thousand miles away or more. Enter the FRG. It is a substitute extended family composed of Army spouses, often wives assigned with their husbands to one duty station. Each FRG will have a slightly different feel and that feel can change over time even at one duty station and definitely changes from one duty station to another. As we are all human and fallible, some FRGs are more well-intentioned than others. But at its core, the FRG steps in and carries out functions that a typical support system would. Meal trains, donations, rides, suggestions on dentists, you name it. If you need it, the FRG should be able to supply it on some level. We all try to help because in essence we are an extended "family" of Army wives and we all understand what it's like to be utterly alone in a completely unfamiliar area. No one else can truly understand our little culture.

The FRG leader called me as soon as she heard about Bill. I picked up the phone and she asked me how Bill was doing. After letting her know what little I knew, she launched into mission mode.

"What do you need?" she asked.

She offered babysitting, a ride to the hospital—whatever I might need. When I let the commander's wife know that I had no way to get our truck home, she sprang into action. By that night, the truck was back at our house. If only they could have helped me figure out what had happened to my husband and whether he was going to be okay or not.

I began bugging a friend who had gone through nursing school with me. After we graduated, she specialized in cardiac intensive care, and since then she had gotten her nurse practitioner degree. She was my go-to for all things heart related. Our text string was a flurry of medical jargon and abbreviations. Bundle branch block, echocardiogram results, troponins, heart rate, chest CT results, pulmonary embolism, pulse pressure, stress test results, cardiac catheterization, oxygen saturation, and on and on. She walked me through his findings from head to toe, and even though she was an expert in the field, she still had no real answers. That worried me. If she couldn't figure out what was happening to Bill, who could?

I hardly ate during the three days Bill was in the hospital. My appetite vanished. My stomach was in knots, and every muscle in my body felt coiled, like a spring wound too tight. I was constantly on edge. I couldn't focus on what the kids needed from me. I just stared into space at the dinner table, numb. The texts and phone calls poured in, one after another, until even responding felt overwhelming. By then, at least, the cardiac events had stopped, and the doctors were starting to talk about discharging him soon. That gave me hope, but not peace.

This was also just a year into Covid. Tensions in the world were beginning to ease but there were still a lot of restrictions. My family and Bill's family were desperate to come and help me and were trying to work it out amongst themselves. Bill's parents were many states away, back on the East Coast. His dad had multiple myeloma so he was considered high risk. Traveling for him was out of the question. His mom was ready to purchase a plane ticket, but my mom convinced her to stay. Bill's dad needed her close, and if she caught Covid while traveling and brought it home, the consequences could be devastating.

Instead, my mom bought the earliest plane ticket she could, and she would be at my house in two days. That was a huge relief, but I still wished I had someone closer. My brother James lived only four hours away in Chicago. When he called and said he was leaving at the end of his workday to come help, I nearly cried with relief.

But that feeling only lasted a few minutes.

My phone rang right after getting off the phone with James. It was my son's school. My stomach, already tight from the stress, now seemed to do flips. It is never good news when the school calls. I answered, and it was the principal on the other end. My son, Thomas, had been exposed to Covid. At the beginning of the school year, the administration had put all the students into small groups of four to five so that they could track and isolate any Covid spread more easily. One of the students in his small group had just tested positive. The protocol was that I would need to pick Thomas up from school and our family would need to isolate ourselves. My heart sank.

I called my brother back to give him the crushing news—Thomas had been exposed to Covid, and we were supposed to isolate. I told him I understood completely if he decided not to come, though I hated saying the words out loud. He was just as disappointed. "I really want to be there," he said, his voice heavy. "But I need to think about it."

An hour later, he called back. His decision was made—he needed to stay home.

I told him I understood. And I did. But that didn't stop the wave of defeat from crashing over me.

There was no cavalry coming.

Why can't anything just be easy?

After what felt like an eternity, the kids and I got the green light to go see Bill. We piled into the car and drove to the hospital, parking in the free garage (a blessing of small community hospitals). We put on masks at the front desk and stated where we were going. We followed a curving hallway to the left and boarded an elevator. Once on the second floor, we walked through the large double doors and checked in with the nurse at the station. She told us his room number. We made our way down the long hallway, glancing at each door, counting down the numbers. His was the very last one.

And there he was—lying in the bed in a hospital gown.

I had never seen him like that before. Not in a hospital. Not as a patient. And certainly not looking scared.

But he did that day.

Normally the kids would be ecstatic to see their father. They would be all smiles and hugs, and I would usually hang back, letting them soak up their moment with him before claiming mine.

But not this time.

This time I was the one to rush to him, and we embraced tightly. We fell into each other's arms and held on tightly. The tears came immediately, and neither of us wanted to let go. We stayed locked in that embrace for several minutes, breathing each other in, anchoring ourselves.

Eventually, our grip loosened. I pulled back and wiped at my face, glancing over at the kids.

They stood frozen, unsure of what to make of the scene. Their parents both wiping away tears. Their dad hooked up to wires, IV drips, and beeping monitors. It was a lot for a child to try to process. Grace had just turned seven and Thomas was only eight.

Grace asked if she could sit on the bed.

I nodded and scooted over to make room. She climbed up carefully and perched beside me, her small frame tentatively pressed against mine, as if unsure whether it was okay to relax.

We visited as long as we could. It was not as long as I wanted it to be. But with two young children who were antsy and a roommate who listened to the television at a deafening level, it was difficult for us to have any quality time. I hoped I would be able to find someone to watch the kids so I could go back and sit with my husband for more than a few minutes.

I smiled to myself, grateful because my neighbors had kindly offered to watch the kids. They'd looked after them before, had grandchildren of their own, and the kids always enjoyed being there. Knowing they were in good hands gave me peace of mind.

As I continued along the familiar curves, the drive began to feel oddly nostalgic. It transported me back nearly twenty years to the early days of dating Bill. Back then, we'd maintained a long-distance relationship because I was in college and he was in the Army. Just a month after we met, the world shifted with the events of September 11th. Life in the military changed overnight, and so did the landscape of our relationship.

Since neither of us could move closer, we made the best of it by driving long distances to see each other or meeting halfway. Sometimes those visits meant twelve or thirteen hours on the road. I remember the butterflies, the sense of anticipation, the joy of seeing him after being apart.

Now, here I was again—driving to see him. Not as my boyfriend this time, but as my husband. Not to a date or a reunion, but to a hospital bed. And still, I cherished the journey. Because he was alive. And that was enough.

After Bill was discharged, I expected him to rebound quickly, given his fitness level. As a nurse, I had taken care of cardiac patients in the hospital, but they had all been in their sixties or older so I assumed Bill's heart would mend faster. We found, however, that even a young person's heart takes a while to heal after injury.

The heart isn't like most muscles. It doesn't get to rest while it heals. It has to keep beating, injury or not. So, recovery takes time. For several weeks after Bill got home from the hospital, he was winded just speaking a sentence. He went from being able to run several miles with ease to getting dizzy before he hit the end of our driveway. If he stood up too long his face became pale and his chest tightened. A month passed. His dizzy spells lessened but continued. He still couldn't drive due to dizziness. I began to wonder if he would ever fully recover. Waiting for an uncertain outcome is one of the hardest things in life. And so, I prayed. I prayed for strength, for clarity, but most of all, for patience. (see Psalm 130:5–6 and Micah 7:7).

Over the next few months we saw emergency medicine specialists, a cardiologist after Bill had worn a heart monitor for two weeks, Bill's primary care doctor, and an endocrinologist. No one could give us an answer as to why this had happened. Our last try was a neurologist. This doctor said he thought, but could not prove, that this had come from the Covid vaccine.

As weeks turned into months, Bill began to heal. He made steady progress, becoming stronger by the day. Eventually, he was able to start driving short distances. With time even walking and then exercising found its way back into his routine. He had fewer and fewer dizzy spells until they faded altogether. We began to breathe easier. It felt like the worst was behind us. We thought our troubles were over. We were wrong.

CHAPTER 5

High Risk

When you pass through the waters, I will be with you; And when you pass through the rivers, they will not sweep over you. When you walk through the fire, you will not be burned; the flames will not set you ablaze.

— Isaiah 43:2 NIV

My dog Toby was a Yorkipoo—that's a Yorkshire Terrier crossed with a small Poodle. Some call it a designer dog. Bill liked to call him an abomination (in jest, of course). Toby was almost fifteen years old at this time and I had gotten him at eight weeks old. His health had been exceptionally good his whole life except for a "trick knee" when he was younger that went away without any intervention. I am so thankful we avoided that costly vet bill!

Toby was a grumpy, cantankerous little dog. He was possessive of his toys and food. By the time we had kids he was already six years old. So by the time they were getting older, he was ancient. Once Toby got tired in the evenings, he would growl if the kids came too close to say goodnight to him (but never bite them). In a nutshell, he could be ornery. But he was one of my best friends. If you're a dog lover, you get this.

In contrast, in the morning he was sweet and pleasant. He loved mornings. He was excited to start the day and it was perhaps the only time of day when he was not grumpy. He would bound up and down the hall with a big grin on his face. He would run and pick up his tennis ball, throwing it in the air a few inches above his head. Maybe part of that excitement was that he knew he would be getting fed right away. He could have stood to lose a couple pounds but I didn't mind. He was my fluffy goofball.

He made the funniest noises—noises that a typical dog would not be proud to make. His growl sounded much like an "Oooooo." He greeted me each day with a teeny, tiny, soft kiss. Each dog has a special place in its owner's heart and my little dog was no exception.

When Toby started acting more lethargic, we took notice. He didn't have the same pep in his step. Then he would start shivering when it was not cold. He would come close to me during the day when I was working at my desk, curl up next to me, and shiver. It seemed out of place, so I called the vet and made an appointment for Toby.

After the X-rays, I sat waiting in the exam room. When the vet entered and asked me to follow him, I wasn't alarmed; this vet often included pet owners in the process, aside from the actual

X-ray itself. I appreciated that about him; he wanted you to be informed.

He pointed out a few structures on the screen, explaining what each one was. Then he paused and tapped his pen on a specific area.

"This is his bladder," he said. "And these… these are bladder stones."

Bladder stones? I can say I was not expecting that to be the cause of Toby's behavior. The treatment? A pretty expensive surgery. I could also wait to see if they would pass, but it had already been a while and the stones were obviously still in the bladder, so it was doubtful they were going anywhere soon. We had to think about our options.

I know for some people electing whether or not to have their dog undergo surgery might be an easy decision. For some people, their dog is their family and they will spare no cost for his health. For others, a dog is a dog and when he gets sick ... well, that's kind of that. My husband and I land somewhere in the middle of those two extremes. And it makes these decisions very difficult. On the one hand Toby was pretty old and had lived a long, full, healthy life. He didn't deserve to be in pain from bladder stones. On the other hand, he could easily live to twenty years old and this was not a disease that would limit his lifespan. It should be a once and done procedure. After some debate, we decided to go ahead with the surgery for Toby.

The day of his surgery, I was to bring Toby in quite early; he would be their first case. I had to leave him and then await the call to come pick him up at the end of the day. I drove the thirty minutes to the vet, anxiously left my dog, and drove back to start my workday. *Might as well work to occupy my mind by working, I suppose. It's better than fretting all day. I hope he's in good hands.*

They called me to come get him around 4 p.m. The surgery had gone well and he was recovering. Very thankful, I hopped in the car with my kids, who had just gotten home from school. We went to pick up our friend.

When we arrived, the girl at the front desk took my payment and stated they would get Toby and our prescription medications for him. She then gave me instructions on how often to give his pain medication, how he should recover, and warning signs to call them back about. Things such as not eating, not going to the bathroom, not waking up, vomiting. It seemed pretty straightforward.

"He will be groggy tonight and it may take until the morning for him to perk up. Give him small quantities of water and food to see how he handles it. There may be blood in his urine for the next few days," the vet tech told me. I was so hopeful things would improve from there on out. Unfortunately, Toby would never be quite the same again.

He seemed to take a long time to recover from anesthesia. He did not want to eat anything that night. I put him on his bed and he didn't leave my room for several hours. They had said he would be lethargic but should be perking up. This little dog typically did not leave my side. I am not exaggerating. Everywhere I went in the house (even the bathroom), Toby absolutely had to follow me. I called him my shadow. As much as I wanted him to be a family dog, he was my dog. That's not to say the family did not enjoy him, or that he did not on occasion enjoy the family, grumpy as he could be. But sometimes a dog just latches onto one person as "his" person. That was Toby and I.

My kids would get frustrated when they went to pet Toby to say goodnight. Inevitably he would growl as they put their hands out close to pet him. He did not bite them; he was just ornery. I would scold Toby and then stroke his head, except he was quiet for me. "Why does he let you pet him and not us?" the children would ask.

"Because I've been his mama since he was a puppy," was all I could say to help them understand. It was a running joke amongst us that Toby was a grumpy old man to everyone but me.

So when I put Toby on his bed and he did not get up to follow me, I was surprised. It was several hours before he stumbled out into the hallway and came into the kitchen. He swayed around like a drunken sailor. He paused and looked at me. He seemed very confused. He got a small drink of water and came closer to me. Then he more or less collapsed on the kitchen floor.

I winced. *That can't be good for his stitches.*

I gave Toby his medication faithfully over the next week. I watched the clock and as soon as I could give it to him, I got out a spoon and put a dab of peanut butter on the spoon and then squished the half tablet into the peanut butter. I offered the spoon to Toby and he gratefully took it. I watched for him to return to his peppy self over the next week. But it just didn't seem to be happening.

He would still shiver from time to time. When he was on his medication, he seemed like he was drunk. We were actually amused and just thought he was high on painkillers. Day after day followed. I had to get a refill of his pain medication because they only gave me enough to last a week. He would sit next to me and shiver from pain. He was slow to get up and go. I knew he was kind of an old man but surely he should have recovered from his procedure after a few weeks?

Looking back, I wish I had taken him back to the vet sooner. I really do. But while I was distracted by Toby's unexplained lack of improvement, something was quietly getting worse for me.

CHAPTER 6

Something Isn't Right

Trust in the Lord with all your heart and lean not on your own understanding; in all your ways submit to him, and he will make your paths straight.

— Proverbs 3:5–6 NIV

After I finally got in to see the neurologist, they were stymied. It wasn't the result I was hoping for. Don't get me wrong, I was really glad to have major diagnoses like multiple sclerosis and ALS (Lou Gherig's disease) ruled out. That was no small thing. But I left the appointment feeling like I was standing in the exact same place as when I walked in. The neuromuscular attacks had been happening for months, and the experts' verdict? A collective shrug. They didn't know what was causing them—and what's worse, they didn't seem to care. Would these symptoms ever stop? Was I supposed to just live with this? It felt like the medical community was looking at my life-altering symptoms and saying, "Meh, don't know, not concerned."

"I know that this is probably frustrating to not have any answers," my neurologist said over a Zoom call on my third appointment with the group. She was young, blonde, very personable, and, most importantly, she actually listened to me. She sat across from me during one visit and wrote down all of my symptoms without judging, without interrupting, and without belittling. That's hard to find in a doctor. Heck, it's hard to find in a human, period. I felt heard, which can be rare when navigating through the medical system.

We were wrapping up our tele visit when she seemed to hesitate for just a moment.

"You should also get an annual EKG and mammogram," she said, her voice a touch more measured. "Some of these disorders can cause some ... irregularities."

I thought that was a little strange, but I had read about heart issues with disorders like muscular dystrophy. Still, something about the way she said it lingered in my mind.

At the same time, I felt a rush of relief. At least whatever was happening wasn't going to leave me unable to walk. I latched onto that reassurance and nodded quickly, ending the call. I had been meaning to speak to my doctor anyway about scheduling a mammogram anyway.

A mammogram uses low-energy X-rays to examine breast tissue. Women don't start getting those screenings until age forty because, statistically, there is a very low chance they will get breast cancer before that age (even before age fifty it is still small) and also because the breasts are denser prior to menopause, which makes irregularities harder to see. I was debating just waiting a year since I was almost thirty-nine and, in a year, I could easily schedule my first screening.

I had, however, just realized that I was at high risk for breast cancer. There are certain calculators that physicians can use to predict how likely a woman is to get breast cancer in her life. Although these are nationally recognized, they are typically something doctors won't calculate unless there is a strong family history or concerning symptoms. I only knew the names of them thanks to my job in insurance. One day, the doctor forgot to send in a patient's score when requesting an MRI. After calculating the patient's score, I wondered what my score might be. After plugging in my numbers, I was a bit surprised to see that my score put me in the high-risk category—just barely. Because of my job reviewing clinical requests for imaging, I knew that meant that my insurance had to cover mammograms and breast MRIs yearly for me starting at age thirty. I was already thirty-eight and could have been getting the imaging for years. I hadn't known.

I had more or less ignored my high-risk result, with my internal debate about telling my doctor ending with a *no, I don't need to*. But now knowing that I was high-risk AND the neurologist wanted me to get a mammogram, I decided it was time to tell my doc. It took a little more convincing than I thought it would.

"Why do you think you're high-risk?" my doctor asked. *Shoot,* I thought; I didn't really have a convincing argument planned and when there's a spotlight on me, I tend to freeze. I searched my brain for a moment, then told her of the neurologist's recommendations, and to boost the likelihood of her agreeing, I also divulged the high-risk information. After I explained my Gail Model risk score, she seemed to give in on the topic.

"OK. The EKG we can do in the office on your next visit. Do you want to schedule the mammogram now or wait until I see you for your next visit?" she inquired. I was relieved that she was willing to do the mammogram. But did I feel like I needed one now? My next yearly visit would be in February, and this was late August. Something nagged at me to schedule it for now.

It was probably a prompting from the Lord, and I probably should have let her know I would get back to her after praying about it. Unfortunately, I decided we could just follow up at my next visit. If I had only known what was growing inside me already. If only I'd scheduled the mammogram just those few weeks earlier, it could have made a drastic difference. But soon enough, I'd figure out on my own that something was not right.

Shortly after the neurologist visit and talking to my doctor, I started having these stabbing pains in my breast. They were short and intense, enough to make me stop what I was doing and wince. After this went on for a few days, I tried to feel the area to see if something was amiss. I felt nothing. I thought maybe it was an abscess.

Earlier that year I had had an abscess in my armpit earlier that year that had to be lanced and drained. That experience was pretty awful and I dreaded the possibility of going through it again. The pains sure felt similar. I knew that a lot of women my age could get cysts or other benign growths in the breast. I did not consider that something more sinister was going on.

A couple weeks went by. The pains kept coming. Then one night, as I was stepping into the shower and felt that same familiar ache, I instinctively prodded the area—and froze.

Is that a lump?

It did feel different than the rest of the tissue, but was it different enough to be ... something, rather than nothing? My mind raced. *What could it be? Did I really feel something? What did my mom say her tumor felt like again? A kidney bean?*

I pressed again. *Does this feel like a kidney bean?*

I didn't want the answer. I wasn't ready for the implications. So I did what felt easiest in the moment: I decided to ignore it. Yes, that's always a productive solution—pretend it doesn't exist, and maybe it won't.

Since Google is a thing now, I began searching for what this could possibly be. I refused to even think the word "cancer" because, being only thirty-eight, it just could not be *that*. My mom first had breast cancer at fifty-nine. Breast cancer was something women near retirement age got. *Although a good friend of ours did have inflammatory breast cancer in her thirties*, my mind nagged. Pushing the thought aside, I found information that said to wait and see if the lump changed size within the next few weeks. *Well, that's close to ignoring it so I'll try that.*

Two more weeks passed. The lump remained, and it did not change size, at least not that I could tell. The pains remained as well. I was still not even sure if I was really feeling a lump or just imagining it. To be honest, part of me still wanted to ignore it. If I did not acknowledge that it existed, it couldn't be anything bad. It couldn't hurt me. It couldn't destroy my life.

But deep in my core, as much as I wished I could avoid this journey, I knew it must be dealt with eventually. I decided to ask my husband what he thought. Maybe a third-party perspective would help affirm or deny the existence of "it."

Bill immediately and decisively said, "Yup, that's a lump. You need to call your doctor." *Darn it.* So rather than calling, because who calls when they can text ... I got on my health portal and fired off a message to my doctor ... a few days later. Triumphantly, I hit send. *There, now I've bought some time before I have to do anything else with this.*

Normally, when I receive a message on my health portal, I get an email alerting me to this new message. For whatever reason, in this instance I did not get any email notifications. And since I didn't want to think about it, I also didn't check. After all, at this same time my best friend from childhood was coming to visit me all the way from Alaska! She was arriving the next day. We only get to see each other every three to five years and she was at the forefront of my mind. The doctor could wait until after our visit.

We had a good time catching up, reminiscing, spending time by the fire, gardening, and having a few drinks. The things best friends do. But in the back of my mind, the lump worried me. I knew a reckoning was coming. My friend stayed for my thirty-ninth birth-day. I watched her making lava cakes with my daughter's help for my birthday dessert choice. Things were good. Until they weren't.

When my best friend left, life resumed its natural course. It occurred to me that I had not received a reply from my doctor regarding finding a lump. That was kind of important, right? So I logged onto my health portal again. There was a message from my doctor all right, that she'd sent two weeks prior! My doctor did not question me or say "I'm sure it's nothing" or make any false promises. I've since learned by speaking to young breast cancer survivors that many young breast cancer patients are pushed to the side in the "let's wait and see" category. Meanwhile, as they are fighting to get the care they deserve, the cancer that is trying to kill them and that is threatening their lives grows. By the time these young women can convince their doctors that something is wrong, the cancer may have had several months of uninhibited growth. Cancer can do a lot within a few months. Trust me, I know.

Cancer works a little like a snowball. At first, the cancer is very small. It can start with just one abnormal cell. As it grows, the number of abnormal cells keeps doubling. By the time something like breast cancer can be felt, it is already about 1–2 cm in size, at least. And that's if you happen to feel it. A lot of people don't. It can double that size in one to three months. Snowball.

To my doctor's credit, she immediately replied to my email (which I didn't see for two weeks) asking if I would rather come in for an exam or just go straight to a mammogram. Thank goodness for that. Once I read her email, I quickly got back to her that I would just like to go right to the imaging. I figured that would be the outcome if I went for a visit anyway, and scheduling a visit would only delay the inevitable imaging I would need in order to get this sorted out. They scheduled me as soon as they could get me in, on October 26th. That was still nearly three weeks away. It seemed so far away. But we have all experienced life after Covid, and one of the side effects seems to be permanently delayed care. That was the earliest they could get me in, so I'd just have to wait.

For the next three weeks I tried to occupy my mind with other things to try to not think about the lump and the pending mammogram. *Everything will be fine.* Or so I thought.

The mammogram did not hurt as I had feared. It was certainly … awkward, though. The technician had to do a lot of coaching. I actually found it quite comical.

"Lean forward. Not that far. Put your left shoulder forward and roll your right shoulder back. Turn your head. Further. Now arch your back. Relax this arm. Okay, put your other arm up and use this handhold. Yes, now try to lean into the machine. Take a small step forward. Hold that pose for a few seconds while I take a picture. Hold your breath. Try not to move. Okay, now you can exhale."

It felt like learning a new dance. An awkward, uncomfortable dance where I didn't know the steps, nothing flowed, and I kept metaphorically tripping over myself. I twisted and turned the way she asked, doing my best to suppress giggles at how ridiculous I felt. The whole experience was strange, but I wasn't especially nervous.

I was convinced the lump would be benign. How could it not be?

CHAPTER 7

The Shock of My Life

May our Lord Jesus Christ himself and God our Father, who loved us and by his grace gave us eternal encouragement and good hope, encourage your hearts and strengthen you in every good deed and word.

— 2 Thessalonians 2:16–17 NIV

The mammogram technician told me to go to the next room over for my ultrasound. I grabbed a white gown with tiny blue diamonds on it and followed another technician to the ultrasound room next door. The sonographer, Megan, squirted the gel on me. Instantly, my mind flashed back to when I was pregnant. That barely-contained excitement of seeing your baby on the screen for the first time. I remembered how the gel used to be icy cold, shocking against already exposed, chilled skin.

But this time, the warmth of it caught me off guard—in the best way. The gel was soothing, and I felt a rush of unexpected gratitude. At some point, they had swapped out the cold stuff for something gentler. A small kindness, but it felt significant. It further bolstered my already high mood, being sure this lump would be nothing and glad I was getting it dealt with.

Megan did what ultrasound technicians do. That is to say, they look at the computer and tell you nothing about what they are doing. They swish their little wand around and click the mouse to take pictures. They type a few things on the images. They save those pictures to your file. They work with incredible speed. Meanwhile you lay there, not sure if they are seeing something completely normal or horribly wrong inside you. You steal glimpses of the screen, but it looks like a fuzzy gray map of a place you've never been and the ultrasound technicians don't give you any hints.

Once done, she said the radiologist was on-site and he would read my images and be right in to explain them to me. She told me to get dressed in the small attached bathroom. The puke-green colored tile was freezing even though I had socks on. I did not sense anything in her tone that concerned me. I dressed quickly, the movement light and almost carefree, then made my way back to the patient bed. I almost smiled. I was glad the hard part was over and was sure the radiologist would come in and say I had a cyst or fibroadenoma: nothing too serious, nothing to worry about.

When Megan reentered, she brought a trainee with her. As soon as they came in, my nonchalant attitude dropped. I immediately sensed the air shift.

Something was off. Neither of these ladies would look at me.

They chose a place to stand, far away from me, stared at the floor or the computer, and looked uncomfortable. I could almost feel the hairs on my neck standing; intuition was warning me already. I tried to brush off the feeling even while I felt like a silent alarm inside me had been activated. While I wrestled with my emotions and tried to figure out if it was all in my head, deep down I no longer wanted the doctor to come in.

When he did, he wasted very little time with formalities and got straight to what he'd come to say. He said, "It is highly likely that this is cancer." And my brain stopped listening.

Silence.

I sat on the uncomfortable exam room bed, clenching and unclenching my jeans. I felt the stiff cotton material in my fingers. Grasping for something to hold onto. The doctor was speaking to me, but his words never reached me. I had seen this special effect in movies before, where the character gets some life-shattering news and the speaker's voice is replaced by a muffled void. I thought it was just for dramatic effect. But I can tell you: it does happen in real life as well.

Except he was actually still talking. Talking about the next steps of pathology, the type of treatment that would follow identification, how far treatment had come. At least, I think that's what he was saying. *He has to be wrong.*

But I couldn't hear it. I couldn't take it in.

Because I hadn't yet grasped the part that mattered most: he was telling me I most likely had cancer.

Cancer.

I had just turned thirty-nine. That couldn't be right. It was impossible.

But I feel fine. It can't be cancer.

Thanks a lot, Google. I had believed Google when my searches told me a breast lump that is painful is not cancer and not to worry because 80 percent of breast masses turn out to not be cancer. *So, this painful lump statistically won't be cancer*, I had told myself. I hadn't had a chance to steel myself for this unexpected news.

I knew Bill would not be expecting it either. I remembered our conversation on the couch a few nights earlier when he had assured me it sounded like a cyst and he had had one before. His doctor told him these things typically go away in a few weeks. I had readily agreed that it was probably nothing. I remembered that conversation with Bill but I honestly don't remember leaving the hospital the day I was told I likely had cancer.

The biopsy, which would confirm or deny that I had cancer, was scheduled for two weeks later. I spent a lot of those two weeks deep in thought. Bill was optimistic. Ever positive, he was convinced it would be benign.

I was not so optimistic. But I didn't want to worry him. So, I put on a brave face—quietly carrying the weight of my fear while letting him hold on to hope.

The day of the biopsy came. Bill took the afternoon off to drive me to my appointment. I appreciated having the physical support of someone with me. Once we arrived, they showed us to the same room where I had had the ultrasound two weeks prior. It's a small hospital so there are only two imaging rooms, but being in the same room was like a haunting reminder from my last visit when the earth dropped from under my feet.

I slipped into the same ugly gown every patient gets, the fabric thin and impersonal. The realization did not escape me that this is how our medical system is as well. I was very nervous.

Mostly about the pain. I can be pretty wimpy when it comes to pain. And I tend to pass out easily during anything painful or invasive. It's just how my body reacts. So yes, I was nervous about the pain and to be honest, also a little about what the result would be.

The doctor breezed in, offered a quick greeting, and gave a brief rundown of the procedure. Then, without missing a beat, he turned to Bill and asked him to wait outside. My heart sank. I had really wanted him there to hold my hand through this and help ground me, like he always did. But Bill didn't budge.

He didn't respond to the doctor. Instead, he turned to me and asked gently, "Is that okay with you?" In that moment, he handed me the power to choose—right in front of the doctor who had looked past me, assuming the decision was already his to make.

I love Bill for moments like that. The small ones that speak volumes.

Ever the people-pleaser, I said, "Yes." But inside I was a bit disappointed.

Once Bill had left, the doctor came around to my right side, where he would be doing the biopsy. I stared at the light. It had one of those coverings over it that are supposed to help calm and soothe you. This was a blue sky with clouds and a few little butterflies. I just wanted to get this over with. I asked God to be with me, and tried to concentrate on Him until the doctor pulled his chair up next to me, interrupting my thoughts. Rather than beginning the procedure, he stopped and waited for me to look at him and then met my eyes.

"You look nervous," the doctor said, his voice calm. I couldn't see his mouth, but the way his eyes squinted told me he was offering a reassuring smile beneath the mask.

Despite the fact that he had kicked my support system out of the room, I did like this doctor. He was jolly and knowledgeable. He was adept at putting me at ease and made it sound like he had done the procedure hundreds of times before. His own wife had undergone a biopsy like this. He and the nurse made jokes to try to cheer me up, and then they commiserated about their long drives into work through bad weather in years past.

"Okay, now I'm going to put the lidocaine in. Little sting here."

I breathed through the pain, just as I had been taught to do for labor pains. *Just focus on long, deep breaths.* It really came in handy and was my go-to whenever I was going through something painful. He commended me for doing well through the injection. I was surprised that it hadn't been that bad.

If you ever deal with high anxiety or need to get through a tough procedure, I highly recommend looking up square breathing—also called box breathing. It's simple, but incredibly effective.

Using ultrasound, he guided the machine that would take the biopsy to where the mass was. This machine resembled a gun.

Luckily all I felt was pressure, thanks to modern numbing medicine. Then he described that he was about to take samples of the tissue. He would get three or four samples. He warned me that the instrument would sound like a gun, and holy cow did it ever! The crack was so loud and sudden, I might have jumped off the bed if he hadn't warned me.

Once he had collected enough samples, it was over. They gave me the usual post-procedure advice: take Tylenol and use an ice pack. I was free to get dressed and leave. The whole ordeal was not nearly as bad as I had anticipated. I was a little sore for a day or two, but honestly—it felt more like the aftermath of a tough workout than anything else.

Three days later I was at my desk working when I decided to check and see if the pathology report was back. To my surprise, it was in my chart, ready and waiting. I opened it up and read: "Ultrasound guided breast biopsy. Suspicious mass at the 9:00 position right breast that corresponds to the patient's palpable abnormality. Specimen received. Final pathologic diagnosis - Invasive ductal carcinoma."

Invasive ductal carcinoma echoed in my head. I stared at the words in disbelief. *How could this be?* I had lived the way you're supposed to in order to *avoid* cancer. I exercised. I ate wholesome, nutritious food. I barely drank alcohol. So why was this happening? The answer would come, but not yet. Not now.

CHAPTER 8

Crisis and Loss

Though he brings grief, he will show compassion, so great is his unfailing love. For he does not willingly bring affliction or grief to anyone.

— Lamentations 3:32–33 NIV

My husband called on his way home that night. After some typical chitchat, he asked how my day was. I felt the urge to spill my guts right then on the diagnosis and be done with the telling part (which I dreaded). But something stopped me.

It felt like an in-person conversation.

I didn't want to tell him over the phone. Maybe I wanted to share the weight of it. To not be alone in that moment of knowing. I wished I could take everything — the ugliness of what I now knew, all my fears, my worries, the dark thoughts—and wrap it into a tight, dense ball.

Then hand it to Bill.

Because somehow, I knew he'd know exactly what to do with it.

"We can talk about that when you get home."

"O-kay," he slowly said, sounding wary.

After we ate dinner and got the kids in bed, we sat on the couch and he asked if I wanted to explain my cryptic statement. I steadied myself, trying to keep my composure. I told him I got the results of my biopsy. "It's cancer." Then I collapsed into his shoulder.

Bill is definitely a guy you want to have around in a crisis. I envy how calm and collected he always is. "Well, we'll get through it, right? We'll get it treated." There was no trace of fear, no hesitation, no hint of sadness or worry. He spoke as if the treatment had already come and gone, as if I were already healed.

I wasn't so sure. I knew I'd have to be the one to go through this. And I'm a wimp, remember?

But in that moment, his certainty became something I could lean on. His strength didn't erase my fear, but it softened the edges—and that was exactly what I needed.

I was suddenly incredibly tired. I had been fairly exhausted since the neuromuscular attacks began. But this was different. This wasn't physical. This was emotional exhaustion, and it ran deeper. Over the next few weeks, it became a pattern. More often than not, I'd head to bed early, drained from the weight of it all.

It wasn't just a phase. It became my new normal; a quiet, heavy fatigue that settled in and stayed like a blanket of heavy snow covering everything.

Just two weeks after learning the news that I had cancer, I made an appointment for Toby at the vet. He still had not gotten better, and he should have felt better by then. I dreaded paying for another surgery after I had just paid for the one to have his stones removed. But I had to do something.

Toby had been having fevers. I had never had a dog have a fever before but I found out when they do, dogs feel incredibly hot to the touch. I had started noticing it occasionally with Toby. I also noticed that his gums and the insides of his lower eyelids were very pale. That's a trick you learn in nursing school that can tell you if someone has anemia. That combined with the fact that he seemed very swollen in the belly made me think his kidneys were failing. By my reasoning, he still had a bladder stone left and it was blocking his ureter, causing fluid to back up into his bladder and forcing his kidneys to shut down since they couldn't pass the fluid out.

It was two days before Thanksgiving and my kids were home from school for break. It was not ideal to have them with me, but I had no other choice. I did what parents always do: We make it work. I loaded the kids into the car and gingerly picked Toby up and set him between the kids. There was no more hopping up into the car for Toby. He could barely walk at that point.

"Mom, Toby is shaking again," my son Thomas said.

I glanced back at the poor pathetic dog situated between my children. His eyes drooped and he sat there shivering, looking miserable. *Shoot.* I ran back inside, grabbed a pill for him, placed it in peanut butter, and went back outside. I quickly gave him the pill, which he took easily.

I gripped the steering wheel and prepared to drive, when a thought occurred to me and I suddenly stopped. I turned around and looked at my children. Their faces were calm. Unbothered. They didn't reflect the deep concern I felt. Not for the dog. Not for the gravity of what might be swirling beneath the surface.

A tug of guilt was nagging at the corner of my mind like a loose thread on the hem of a shirt. I hadn't told them about my diagnosis yet, either. And sitting there in the quiet stillness of the car, I realized how much I was holding. For all of us.

I thought quickly, trying to simplify adult subjects for my kids. "Toby is pretty sick, guys. The vet may not be able to fix him. He may have to give Toby a special medicine that causes him to go to sleep…forever."

I hated saying the words even as I was forming the sentence. I did not want to think of the possibility that this was my last day with Toby. But I knew it was, indeed, a possibility and one my children needed to be aware of and prepared for. I did not want this to come out of the blue for them. I couldn't let it blindside them. I suppressed the thought that I'd need to do the same for my own medical treatment soon. *One thing at a time.*

With our previous dog, we had done things differently. We knew it was his last day when we took him to the vet, but the kids were so young we did not prepare them. We told them to say goodbye, but they didn't understand we meant say goodbye forever. They were never able to process the first dog's death and did not get over it. I hoped this time would go more smoothly. But then, did I actually want them to witness it? The prospect seemed morbid.

When we got to the vet, I walked in slowly with Toby. Or rather, *he* walked slowly and I matched his pace; something I'd needed to do more and more often recently on our walks. Once we got into a room, I tried to comfort Toby and noticed he was on fire. Like, feverishly hot. *Poor thing.* The vet came and briefly spoke with me and quickly decided he wanted to get some labs. They picked up Toby and whisked him away temporarily. It surprised me how quickly he came back with the results of the labs.

"So, his white blood cells are very high and his red blood cells are very low. I'd like to do an X-ray."

He handed me the printout of Toby's labs from his bloodwork. I was shocked to see his white blood cells were twice what they should have been and his red blood cells were a third of what they should have been. I agreed to the X-ray. Again, it was not long before they were back. The vet looked crestfallen. He didn't mince words. His expression said it all before he even opened his mouth—and when he did, the truth came out plain and heavy.

"He has a splenic mass. I'll show you if you want to come back." He gestured toward the back, where the equipment was.

With no time to process, I scooped Toby into my arms (he was too weak now, even a short walk left him spent) and followed the vet to the back of the building. He kindly showed me the images from just two months prior, when we had found the bladder stones, and you could not see the mass at all. Not even a shadow. Now, it was unmistakable: a softball-sized mass on the spleen.

It had grown so much in just two months.

The thought that *my* cancer could be capable of doing the same thing clawed at the edges of my mind.

But I wouldn't let it in.

I refused to give that fear any power.

Not right now. Right now, this terrible reality had to be dealt with.

The vet went through the options, which were limited. I could try the vet school in Indianapolis where they might be able to do emergent surgery to possibly extract the mass, or I could humanely end his life. My soul felt crushed under the weight of this decision. This dog had been with me for almost fifteen years. He was my child before I had children. He was with me through all eight of Bill's deployments. He was a part of me.

I knew what had to be done, and I hated to do it. But looking at Toby I felt a slight comfort that his troubles would be over. He'd spent the last two months feeling miserable. He was not himself anymore. Often in pain, not eating or drinking as much, hardly able to walk at times, with frequent fevers. I guess the writing had been on the wall but I just didn't see it. His life force had been drained away from him as the tumor ate more and more of his precious red blood cells.

I knew I had to release him from this state. With a heavy heart, I looked at the vet and told him our decision.

I called my husband to give him the bad news and see if he could pick up the kids, so I could attend to this terrible business.

But he was stuck and couldn't come.

Now I had to decide: should I come back after the holiday, or do it right then and there? Every part of me wanted to delay. I wanted to scoop Toby up and run away with him—cuddle him until his time came gently, in my arms.

I told the vet we'd be back the next day. I didn't want the kids to see it. I wasn't ready for them to carry that image.

But as I was leaving, the ladies at the front desk gently stopped me. They offered to watch the kids, to distract them with a sweet puppy who happened to be there. Their kindness opened a door I hadn't expected. I felt like that could work.

I paused, heart aching, then turned back to the vet.

"Can we do it now?" I asked.

I took Thomas and Grace into the exam room and looked them in the eyes. I told them that Toby was too sick for the vet to fix him and since he was suffering, the vet would have to give Toby medicine that would make him sleep and pass away peacefully. They were tearful but astonishingly seemed to accept this fact with no arguments. I had them say their goodbyes and told them they could go play with the puppy in the lobby. Within a few minutes, they were completely distracted.

The vet and tech solemnly went about the unpleasant task. First by giving the sedative and then the euthanasia medicine. Their movements were quiet and respectful, but to me, it all felt impossibly loud. Final.

And then he was just, gone. As I sat there, I felt a sharp ache bloom in my chest—like something had been ripped away from inside me. Watching Toby go, knowing my loyal buddy was really gone… it shattered something deep. I cried harder than I have in decades.

The kids were crushed. They cried a little, their faces crumpled in grief. They were surprised at how alive Toby still looked. And that made it even harder to understand. Harder to accept. Being seven and eight years old, their experience with death was limited and they asked me if I was sure he was dead.

"Are you sure he isn't just sleeping?" Thomas asked

I assured him that Toby was not just sleeping and we would be getting his ashes back, just as we had with our other fourteen-year-old dog Piper that had died two years prior. A few weeks later we did get his ashes, along with his paw pressed into clay. I still keep it next to my bed. A small, quiet reminder of the love that never left.

To my surprise, the kids moved on quickly. Not out of coldness, but in that beautifully baffling way children do, which is appropriate for their ages. They would digest their grief in bits and pieces over the weeks to come but it would be under the surface, rather than a constant visible grief.

"Can we go to the trampoline park now?" one of them asked, not long after we said goodbye to Toby. I blinked, stunned for a moment. But then I nodded. They deserved some joy after the heaviness of the day. We went to the trampoline park even though all I wanted was to go home, crawl into bed, and disappear under the weight of my own heartbreak

That night the house seemed too quiet. I stared at the empty dog bed next to my side of our bed, that small, silent space now unbearably loud in its absence. The night felt darker. My head hurt, and again I was tired. Selfishly, I was also sad that my best animal friend wouldn't be by my side for my own cancer journey, which hadn't even begun yet.

The darkness I felt wasn't just mine—it's in the world, in all the sin, sadness, and confusion that surrounds us.

I was thankful, deeply thankful, that I had found God before the storm hit. I was thankful I had already found God for the hard times. The rock that is higher than I (see Psalm 61:2).

Two weeks later I dreamed of Toby. In my dream, he was in Heaven. He was swimming in a river with many children: Laughing, joyful children who played with him like he was their beloved companion too. He was so happy; his mouth wide open with a big smile (as much as a dog can smile). When I woke up, tears sprang up in my eyes immediately and I was overwhelmed, like I had actually been there with him, just for a moment. I hope that dream was a glimpse of what he's really doing in Heaven.

I still wished he was here with me. I probably always will.

But knowing he was *that* happy—even just in a dream—brought me a peace I didn't know I needed.

I didn't know it yet, but someone would be with me throughout my journey. Someone to commiserate with. Someone who had already walked through this darkness and come out the other side. Someone who could truly understand. Who could sit with me in the heaviness, without needing to fix it.

I didn't know it yet…but I wasn't going to be alone.

CHAPTER 9

Statistically Unlikely Events

Her children arise and call her blessed.
— Proverbs 31:28 NIV

When you learn you have cancer, your dance card is suddenly quite full. Suddenly, your calendar overflows with doctor's appointments, scans, consults, and procedures. There are so many doctor's appointments to go to. You meet all kinds of specialists: Oncologists, radiation oncologists, surgeons, physical and occupational therapists, nurse navigators, nutritionists, pharmacists, geneticists… the list seems endless. In what feels like no time at all, they become part of your everyday vocabulary. You quickly learn who they are, what they do, and how each one fits into this strange, new world you never asked to enter.

Another very unpleasant part of cancer is insurance. We have good insurance, or at least I thought we did. I did not realize how many doctors were NOT in our insurance plan until I began getting bills from the visits. When I called my insurance company, they stated that the doctors were out of network and I would need to pay for my half of their fees.

How can someone be out-of-network when they're literally in the same building—just one door down—from a provider who *is* in-network?

Same practice. Same hallway. Same logo on the wall.

I have no idea how that works. But apparently, that's how it is.

We are rural, so network providers for us may be well over an hour away. The bills began stacking up. I tried in vain to work it out with my insurance company.

Up until this point, I had always been able to call and get any bumps in the road with insurance cleared up. I had successfully argued out of bills due to incorrect codes, incorrect doctor identification numbers, places of service, or type of service listed. Full disclosure, this is what I did for a living at the time (and still do). So you'd think I could easily handle this new challenge.

But this time, I couldn't seem to make any headway. My mind, once sharp and confident when it came to these things, felt foggy. Unfocused. I couldn't think straight anymore.

When I tried to argue with the insurance reps on the phone, I'd end up emotional—tears welling up before I could even finish my case. Eventually, I'd hang up, overwhelmed and defeated, still reeling from the cold, unhelpful responses of the staff on the other end.

One night I opened a bill for the surgeon I had seen. I already had a consult. I already had a surgery date. I'd even received my prep instructions.

But staring at the bill, I realized she wasn't in our network. Panic crept in. I knew that trying to find a new, in-network surgeon and securing an appointment would delay my care by weeks—maybe even a month or more. And I knew what that could mean. My cancer could keep growing. It could spread. I had just seen with my own eyes what happened with my dog's cancer a few days prior. Toby's cancer had gone from nonexistent to the size of a grapefruit in two months. Two months. My cancer had already been there over three.

I had even noticed my lump felt like it was getting bigger. I was still reeling from having to put down our dog. My cancer was growing, maybe spreading to other places in my body. I no longer trusted my body. It felt like enemy territory; danger could be lurking anywhere, lying in ambush.

My hands were still trembling when I opened the next envelope. It was a letter denying my intermittent FMLA. The reason? A lack of notes from my doctor. That was the moment it all became too much.

How could I fight cancer while also fighting my insurance company and juggling endless paperwork?

I broke down at the table. Just started crying.

It wasn't like me. But that night, I couldn't hold it in anymore

Bill comforted me. He said he would take time off from work to help me get everything sorted out. I can't describe the relief I felt.

My brain had turned to mush since the diagnosis. I couldn't keep track of who was in or out of our insurance network anymore, and even basic paperwork felt impossible to navigate. And true to his word, he did it.. He took nearly a full day off work to call different points of contact, find information, and persuade insurance.

He was the help I desperately needed in that moment.

Later, I called my insurance and asked for a case manager. They didn't sound thrilled about the request but eventually, they assigned one. And having her changed everything.

She became a lifeline. She directed me to the right doctors (ones actually in-network) and stepped in on my behalf when claims came through stamped *"out of network."* She made sure the claims department understood: I had an exception, because we lived in such a rural area.

It took a couple of months, but eventually, the insurance situation got sorted out.

I even got approved for FMLA. Honestly, I'm still not entirely sure how—it's such a complicated mess—but either I or the doctor managed to do enough of the right things at the right time.

God was working in the little details.

The other complication was telling the kids about my diagnosis. I knew that they would be scared if I used the word "cancer," so I debated whether to use it. After a lot of back-and-forth, I decided not to. One night when Bill was away for business, I figured I would rip off the proverbial band-aid.

"So, guys," I began carefully. "I have a lump inside me that the doctors don't want there. So they are going to take it out. I'll have to have surgery in a couple months."

No reaction. They just accepted this and said "Okay" as if I had said I was going to put gas in the car next week. They went right back to eating their breakfast.

I was astounded. *Was that really just that easy?* I thought. I had anticipated questions, fear, something? I had not anticipated nothing.

But as the days passed, I couldn't shake the feeling that what I'd shared hadn't been enough. We live in a very small town—where news travels faster than you'd think. When Bill had his heart attack, I'd told *one* teacher. One. And within a week, the story had spread through the entire school and beyond.

I kept imagining a scene I couldn't bear: another kid at school blurting out, "I heard your mom has cancer." And then my child, confused and blindsided, coming home with wide eyes, asking if it was true. I'd have to fess up, not in my words or on my terms, but in damage control.

That didn't feel right. I knew I had to do better. For them, and for me.

Not wanting to have that story play out, I figured I needed to use the word "cancer" somehow. I dreaded their reactions. Again, I chose a time when I was alone with them. I seized my opportunity when Grace asked about my upcoming surgery again.

"Well," I said, gently choosing my words, "they have to cut the cancer out. And once they do that, they'll look at it to decide what my treatment will be."

As I spoke, my mind flashed back to when my own mom had told me about her breast cancer diagnosis eleven years earlier. I remembered how carefully she had chosen her words too, trying to protect me from the full weight of it, just as I was doing now with my own children. I had stood up and hugged her then, in what was, for me, a rare moment of openly showing emotion. I've never been great at expressing my feelings, especially not the heavy ones, but I remember wanting her to know I was there with her. Now, it was my turn to be on the other side of that conversation.

Their silence went on too long for comfort. For an uneasy moment they both stared at me with open mouths. Thomas suddenly shrieked, "You didn't tell us you have *cancer!*"

Both kids sprang from their seats and rushed to wrap their arms around me. Their little bodies pressed tightly into mine, their embrace full of fear and love and a need to protect that they didn't quite know how to express. I wished I did not have to put them through this. That I could protect them. I know God wishes the same for us.

They didn't take it as easily as they had with my first, vague explanation. This time, the weight of the word "cancer" landed. But still, they rebounded more quickly than I expected. Kids have a remarkable way of absorbing hard things and letting joy and normalcy back in.

In the coming months, I translated as best I could all the things that would happen to me to my kids. I made sure to break it down into simple words and not elaborate. I did not want them to know all the bad things that might happen. I didn't give them statistics or go into the possibilities that were plaguing my brain in silence. They did not need to worry about what ifs – what if it doesn't work, what if it spreads. I told them about each treatment and what the doctors hoped it would do.

Thomas and Grace did have some behavior issues at school that academic year that were uncharacteristic. I was not sure whether it was just them being kids or if it was related to their parent's recent health concerns. Either way, we decided to give them extra grace. We didn't discipline them that year the way we normally would have for what we took as their young minds trying to make sense of big, scary changes.

About a month after my cancer diagnosis, I was talking to my mom on the phone.

"So, where was your lump?" she asked. Her voice was steady, but there was something in her tone. She was trying too hard to be causal and was too pointed. It made me pause. I felt a flicker of unease, as if she already knew something I didn't. The question wasn't casual. It carried weight, and I sensed it was leading somewhere I wasn't ready to go.

I explained that it was on the right side near my armpit.

"Hmm. Funny thing, I had a mammogram last week that found a suspicious spot in the same place. What Bi-Rads number did they give yours?"

"Five," I reminded her.

The Bi-RADS scale is a system that radiologists use to help determine how suspicious a finding, like a lump or mass, is when seen on an imaging test like a mammogram or ultrasound. The scale goes from 0 to 5. A lower number, like 1 or 2, usually means everything looks normal or very likely to be harmless. But the higher the number, the more concerned the doctor is that it could be cancer. A 5 means it's highly likely to be cancer, and more testing or a biopsy is usually recommended.

"They gave me a five as well," she said plainly.

I felt like time stood still for a moment. The air seemed to get sucked out of the room. It felt like a lifetime before I could process the news. It was so unfair!

My mother had already been through cancer. She had beaten it. She endured every awful treatment they threw at her. Chemotherapy had stripped so much from her—it made her faint, made her vomit, made her waste away. It drained her strength, stole pieces of her that took years to rebuild. And yet, she did everything right. She took the medications they said would help prevent it from returning. She had been cancer-free for eleven years. Eleven years! It felt so unjust. How could it come back now, after everything she had already been through?

I could tell she was disappointed, but my mother has a spirit that cannot be crushed. Long before it was common to see women in positions of power, she had already shattered ceilings: serving as a CNO, a CEO, a VP, and a director of national operations. And she did it all while raising our family, with my father faithfully by her side. I don't remember her ever taking a single sick day throughout my entire childhood. She worked holidays, taking on-call duties without complaint.

She is the smartest, toughest person I know. She overcame a childhood marked by hardship—an alcoholic father and a mother who may have struggled with some sort of narcissistic personality disorder. And yet, my mom built an extraordinary life. Now, facing cancer for the second time, she was shaken, but not fazed. Her bravery was unwavering. She stood tall, resolved to face this monster again. And in watching her, I found courage of my own.

Just before my mom's cancer recurrence, my oncologist ordered a genetic test. The nurse explained it was standard protocol since I was so young, and reassured me not to worry—only 5 to 10 percent of tests come back positive for the breast cancer gene (BRCA).

Well, guess what? I was part of that 5 to 10 percent. Statistically unlikely, yet somehow, here I was.

It felt like every time I turned around, I was handed another one-in-a-million card. Another blow that defied the odds. And as it turned out, this wouldn't be the last time. There were more statistically unlikely events waiting for me.

By now I was basically on a maintenance program with the neurologist. Even if I wasn't, my nervous system had taken a backseat to the cancer. That had become the priority, and neurology appointments were no longer top of mind. I updated my chart with the neurology team, telling them that I had been diagnosed with breast cancer, and then I moved on without giving it much more thought.

At my next visit, though, they told me something unexpected: they were now diagnosing me with paraneoplastic syndrome. It's rare—only about 8 percent of people with cancer develop it. Essentially, it's an abnormal immune response triggered by the presence of cancer cells. My body, in trying to fight the cancer, had become confused. My antibodies and white blood cells were mistakenly attacking healthy cells in my nervous system, which explained the strange neurological symptoms I had been having.

They said there wasn't a treatment unless the symptoms became severe, in which case they could try an infusion. Otherwise, the best hope was that once the cancer was treated and gone, my immune system would settle down on its own.

Yet another rare diagnosis. Another medical anomaly. It was starting to feel like my body was collecting them.

Even though they couldn't get my blood to match any of the known markers for paraneoplastic syndrome, they felt the diagnosis was accurate. I was actually relieved to have the mystery solved—it was validating to finally have an explanation.

I thought of my oncologist who had blown off the idea. I had told her that the neurologists had collected my blood to test in a panel because they suspected this syndrome. "No, you don't have that. Do you know how low the chances would be?"

I suppose the odds don't always determine the outcome.

I didn't focus on any of that, though. My focus was more on the pain. The twinges of pain got more intense, more frequent, and had started to spread to under my arm. I did not like where I thought this was going.

CHAPTER 10

The Balrog

"Nevertheless, I will bring health and healing to it; I will heal my people and will let them enjoy abundant peace and security."

— Jeremiah 33:6 NIV

Once I had weathered the crushing blow of my cancer diagnosis and finally cleared the exhausting hurdles with insurance, it was time to turn my attention to treatment. My team was optimistic because we caught it early. That was a huge relief. Finding it early often means you can avoid chemotherapy altogether, and I clung to that hope tightly.

I had watched my mom battle through chemo over a decade ago, and I remembered every detail. It drained her, both physically and emotionally. It made her feel truly awful. That experience had etched itself into my memory, and I wanted no part of it.

To me, chemotherapy felt like the Balrog from *The Lord of the Rings*—a massive, terrifying beast hidden in the depths, one that you avoid at all costs. If you're not a Lord of the Rings fan, just know: it's the thing even the wizard doesn't want to mess with.

First up would be surgery. I was not nervous at all for this part; rather, I was excited to be getting this killer cut out of me as soon as possible. The week before my surgery, I definitely noticed that the lump was starting to look and feel bigger. This didn't concern me too much though, because in a few days, I was getting it OUT. It would be gone, for good.

The morning of the surgery, I woke up in a good mood. Not even the gnawing hunger from having to fast overnight could get me down. I couldn't wait to get the process started. I chose matching shades of lavender and purple from my head to my toes. Comfy jogging pants, a warm, loose-fitting sweatshirt. I hoped the clothes would be easy to get back on after my surgery. We got the kids on the bus, said a prayer with my parents, and set off for the hospital. I thought I would get admitted to surgery pretty quickly. Little did I know that they had some torture planned for me first.

First up in the house of horrors was a little procedure called "needle localization." Before surgery, they had to insert a wire into the tumor to help guide the surgeon. First came the lidocaine injection, which I was told would numb the area. But, as my nurse explained with a sympathetic wince, "some tumors soak up the lidocaine because they're so vascular." Lucky me—mine was one of those. That meant most of the numbing medication didn't stay where it was needed, and the pain was significant.

My nerves ramped up when they mentioned that the regular doctor wouldn't be doing the procedure. Instead, a fill-in doctor came in...only to fumble around looking for supplies. She couldn't find a face shield, which didn't exactly inspire confidence. We had to wait what felt like hours while they searched other rooms for one. Once she was finally suited up and I was prepped, the real ordeal began.

The only thing that made the experience even remotely bearable was my nurse. She kindly held my hand the entire time. I focused all my energy on not crushing her fingers, and somehow, that distraction helped me ride out the pain.

After I was good and skewered, it was time for a mammogram. They really have to squish your tissue for these. Why would they ever do something so horrid to a now-tender area, you might ask? Well it's because they need to make sure the wire had actually hits its target (the cancer) and not some innocent, healthy tissue nearby. The first machine we went to did not cooperate. My nurse apologized as she tried to get the beast to load whatever computer program it needed to run. About ten unsuccessful minutes later, she said we'd have to go to the alternate machine across the hall.

At this point, with the amount of pain I'd just endured, and having not eaten since dinner the night before, I started to feel a little sick. I tried to ignore it, but it wouldn't go away. Then came the slow, creeping realization of what was happening—what *always* seems to happen to me in these situations. This has been a recurring theme in my life: no food, plus a medical procedure, usually equals fainting.

Ever since that first time I drove myself to the doctor for a routine vaccine—only to promptly faint at the check-out window—I've learned to recognize the signs of an impending fainting spell. The cold sweat. The queasiness. The white noise slowly overtaking my ears.

Great, I thought. *Now I'm going to faint.*

"Can I sit down? I'm not feeling well," I managed to get out just as the white noise roared in my ears and my vision began to tunnel. I knew from experience that staff much prefer a heads-up over having someone crash to the floor like a sack of potatoes.

And believe me, I've learned that the hard way. Fainting without warning doesn't just cause a scene—it causes pain. I've woken up with bruised hips and a scuffed-up face from fainting episodes before. It's like someone hits a reboot button on your consciousness and you wake up after you've been in a fight unknowingly.

I also knew from experience, once you alert the medical staff, the flapping begins. By which I mean they hustle around and fret over you and look very anxious. Usually they call for help. That's what my nurse did this time. I got seated and slumped over, taking deep breaths to try to stay conscious. Once they have a helper, someone usually gets a cold cloth to put on the victim or some smelling salts, possibly water or juice to drink. They got a cold cloth this time. The cold cloth on the back of the neck always seems to help.

When my breathing returned to normal and I could see again and all the other symptoms faded, it was finally time to get squished where I had just gotten stabbed. I made it through the mammogram after the near-faint. Then they took me into another room to await the next torture device. Luckily, they did let Bill come in at that point. I'm not sure if it was because I had almost fainted and they wanted more eyes on me (or help catching me should I try it again) or if he would have been welcomed by then anyway. Either way, it was nice to have my support by my side again.

The next step was the dye injection. In this process, a radioactive tracer dye is injected near the tumor. The body will naturally sweep the dye to the sentinel lymph nodes. This dyes the nodes bright blue or green, making them jump out at the surgeon so he or she can easily remove them for sampling.

The radiopharmacist came and explained the procedure to us. She already seemed to be apologizing for how much it was going to hurt. She said most people say it feels like burning. I won't lie, it wasn't pleasant. But it also wasn't as bad as the wire placement had been. If you've ever been stung by a fire ant, it felt like that. I took deep breaths and tried to blow out the discomfort. This didn't seem to last too long.

That finally wrapped up the horror show. Now we were able to go back to the surgical area and get prepped. They gave me a lavender gown to wear and purple nonskid socks. I took it as a good omen. I'd worn lavender and purple that day, too. Surely that had to mean something.

The gown, I have to say, was one of the most impressive things I've ever seen in a hospital setting. It had a built-in heating system. I'm not kidding—you could choose how warm you wanted to be, and a fan blew toasty air through little vents inside the fabric. Why are surgical areas always approximately the temperature of a walk-in freezer? No idea. But I cranked that baby all the way up.

After a few minutes, I was warm and snug. So warm it almost made up for the stabbing, squishing, and wire-jabbing that came before. Almost.

The surgery was ... well, I have no idea how it was because I was asleep. Remind me to thank God for whoever discovered anesthesia. It felt like they wheeled me into the operating room and I was immediately getting the best sleep of my life, and then they rudely kept asking me to wake up back in my room. I didn't want to wake up. I munched goldfish crackers and sipped Sprite. I heard the surgeon say something about two lymph nodes. I assumed that they took two lymph nodes out for testing.

They handed me an ice pack, told me I could get dressed, and then more or less hurried us out the door. Whew. I felt a wave of relief wash over me. It was gone!

I truly believed that from here, it would be smooth sailing. I had no idea just how much I would need God for the next part of the journey.

CHAPTER 11

Spiraling

But if from there you seek the Lord your God, you will find Him if
you seek Him with all your heart and with all your soul.

— Deuteronomy 4:29 NIV

Turns out, the two lymph nodes the surgeon was talking about were two positive nodes. They took out four nodes, and out of those, two had cancer in them. Fifty percent. That was a pretty devastating blow.

And the cancer inside was macrometastases rather than micrometastases, which just means there are more cancer cells (read: bad).

As if that weren't enough, the tumor itself had doubled in size. My first imaging had measured it at 1.4 cm, or roughly the size of a peanut. The sample the lab received was 3.1 cm. This is the size of an average strawberry. For days after getting that news, anxiety had me in a chokehold. I couldn't stop myself from Googling every medical term on my pathology report. I spiraled through rabbit holes, comparing statistics, outcomes, recurrence rates. I devoured article after article, trying to predict my future from charts and numbers.

To say the stats were discouraging is putting it mildly.

The margins around my tumor had also been closer than they normally like to get. Surgeons like margins to be about 2 mm wide. My surgeon told me that she had cut as deeply as she could without cutting into my muscle. The margin (the space between the tumor and the edge of what was removed) on the lab report was less than 1 mm. This is about the width of a pencil tip or a credit card. That tiny sliver was all that stood between me and stage 4 breast cancer—when the disease breaks free from its original site and begins invading surrounding tissues like muscle.

Stage 4 is as high as the scale goes.

Thankfully, my cancer was ultimately classified as stage 2B. But knowing how close I came… that haunts me sometimes. And the anxiety it created in me started a cascade.

In the following weeks while at work, I picked up and put down my phone hundreds of times. I was checking for reports, Googling prognosis, and looking for notes from my oncologist with a compulsive force. Whirlwinds of thoughts came in and swirled around my head without ceasing, sweeping my peace up along with their tempest.

It began to remind me of another time when God spoke to me in the midst of my fear. The Covid-19 pandemic had just hit. I, like millions of other Americans, was working from home. Isolating, as it we called it. Like others, I was consumed with the news. I obsessively scrolled news feeds to see where and how badly the virus was spreading, as if that would make me feel better.

As I reached for my phone for the hundredth time one morning, I immediately heard a clear voice say, "What will you find there?"

As if I had already thought about the words ahead of time, I responded equally fast with, "Bad news."

The voice continued right away, "What will you find in me?"

I knew the answer just as easily again. "Good news."

A calm relief had washed over me and I put my phone down. God's voice was right, of course. With that brief exchange, the Father was wrapping His loving arms around me and gently redirecting my gaze back to Him. He wants to do the same for you. He wants to give you His peace and good news.

Friends, we will never find true peace in this world. It just isn't going to happen. Our only lasting peace is found in Him. He calms the storms of our minds and hearts. As it says in Philippians 4:7: "And the peace of God, which surpasses all understanding, will guard your hearts and your minds in Christ Jesus."

Remembering that encounter helped soothe my soul. Which I would desperately need for the days ahead.

A few days later, I sat waiting in yet another doctor's office for yet another appointment. My husband was with me. This was THE appointment. The one where the oncologist would lay out a plan. We had tested me for the BRCA mutation and learned I did indeed have a mutation on my BRCA2 gene. This is a genetic mutation that puts you at higher risk for breast and ovarian cancers.

We had done surgery and tested lymph nodes. We had gotten the Oncotype score, an important piece of the puzzle. This score helps predict how likely the cancer is to return. My doctor had all this information, along with my age and history, at her fingertips to determine what she thought was the best course of action for me.

My oncologist, Dr. Dowell, entered the room with a nurse behind her, wheeling a computer cart. The doctor was slight and wiry, probably only about ten years older than me, and brimming with a quiet confidence. We had first met shortly after my diagnosis at a new patient visit in early December. I had already had some time to "come to terms" with the cancer, and I was somewhat looking forward to the appointment because it would mean a clear set of steps and I would learn what to expect next. When the visit was coming to an end, Dr. Dowell paused and then asked something that surprised me. As the appointment wrapped up, Dr. Dowell paused, then asked something I didn't expect:

"Are you religious?"

I didn't think doctors still asked that kind of thing, but I was glad she had. I nodded. "Yes… why?"

She gently glanced me up and down. "You just seem like you have the peace of the Lord on you," she said. "So I had to ask."

I was stunned. I *had* felt the peace of the Lord—but was it really that visible? How could she tell?

It was yet another small God coincidence in my life.

Dr. Dowell started talking about my case and going over all the data we had on me. With all the information she had, I learned that things were not any clearer. Even my doctor had been on the fence. Every result was just over or just under the "threshold" of where she would typically recommend chemotherapy. My case was as borderline as you could possibly get. She had even consulted the main geneticist on their research team at the big city university about my case and he came up with the same conclusion. "It's just a patient choice at this point," she quoted him as saying.

"If you asked four oncologists, you'd probably have two who recommend chemotherapy and two who don't." Then she said the words I had been dreading since the get-go: "I'm recommending chemotherapy."

My heart was crushed. I was stunned into silence. All I could think was, *I can't do chemotherapy; I won't do it.*

With my mind racing, I could not think of any questions. Besides, I wasn't going to do the chemotherapy, so why ask questions? Luckily, my husband Bill was smart enough to know we had to ask at least one question.

"What are the side effects?" he asked, to the point. He was always level-headed, good in an emergency. I could count on him. Little did I know how much I would have to count on him in the coming months.

The doctor listed off the side effects. Nausea and hair loss were the main two. She said most women are disappointed that they don't lose any weight at all. "The medications are so good now," she said, "that we don't let patients get too nauseous and stay they the same weight." I tried to give her the amused smile I knew she was hoping for. It ended up more like a worried little twitch at the corner of my mouth. Not that it mattered much—this was a post-COVID world, and everything in healthcare was still happening behind a mask anyway.

I knew she was telling the truth—as she understood it. Probably as someone who had never been through chemotherapy herself. But I knew a different side of chemo. I remembered watching my mom endure it. She lost a lot of weight. She lost strength. She struggled. It drained her. It was not just a little nausea. What I saw her go through … I knew I wasn't up for that.

I asked for the weekend to think it over and pray about it. "Of course," she said. But I knew in my heart that I'd already made the decision. I was too scared to do it. I just wanted to postpone telling her no.

That weekend I spent a lot of time in quiet reflection. I prayed almost nonstop. I tried to be still so that I could hear God's voice. After Friday night, all day Saturday, and more than half the day Sunday, I hadn't heard anything. I didn't feel anything. I hadn't had a dream or come across any coincidences from the universe. I was just about to throw in the towel and stick with my compulsion. I would stay the course I had picked and tell my doctor no thank you to the chemotherapy.

I was washing the dishes, standing and looking out at our beautiful backyard with the view of the woods. It was February so I could see far down into the hollow and up the other side. It was my favorite time of year for looking out that window. It looks like we live high up in the mountains when the leaves are gone, even though in reality, we're just perched on a small hill.

Then suddenly, I received exactly what I needed.

A small voice whispered, *"For such a time as this."*

I knew instantly what the voice was referring to. And I knew, without a doubt, that I had to call my doctor.

CHAPTER 12

Hearing that Still, Small Voice

*"Whoever belongs to God hears what God says. The reason you do
not hear is that you do not belong to God."*

— John 8:47 NIV

To be clear, I'm well aware that in our society, people who
say they hear voices are often labeled as crazy. Honestly,
earlier in my life, if someone had told me that God had
spoken to them, I probably would have raised an eyebrow, too.
I may not have all my marbles (who really does?), but the voice
I'm referring to isn't some booming sound from the clouds or a
hallucination. It's the still, small voice of God—the quiet prompting of the Holy Spirit. Jesus compared the Holy Spirit to a breeze.
Where does it come from? Where is it going (see John 3:8)?

It's not easy to explain. This kind of hearing comes through
prayer, time in Scripture, stillness, and a heart that's open and listening. It takes discernment. Some people never experience this

kind of communication from God; it's just not how He chooses to speak to them.

All I can say for myself is this: when the voice speaks to me, it comes faster than my own internal dialogue. Before my brain can even process what I'm thinking, the words are just there. It's not something I'm manufacturing—it feels placed, not produced.

And something I hold tightly to is this: the Spirit will never say anything that goes against the Bible. That's one way I know it's not just my own wishful thinking or wandering thoughts.

I prayed over and over for many years to hear from God. To me, He speaks very seldom. And the few times I have hear from Him? I hold those moments close. I cherish them.

"For such a time as this" comes from the book of Esther. I would highly recommend reading it. It is one of my favorite books of the Bible. It's like a suspenseful movie unfolding as you read. There are plot twists right and left. It's the only book of the Bible that does not mention God. Much like life, it's up to the reader to interpret God's presence and divine intervention amongst the pages.

In Esther 4:14, Esther's uncle Mordecai is asking her to do something risky. Something that could get her killed. But it's out of desperation that he asks her, as the Jews are facing extinction via a murderous executive order. To paraphrase, he tells her, "If you do nothing, deliverance for our people will come from somewhere, but you and your father's house will perish. And who knows whether you have not come to the kingdom for such a time as this."

It's about destiny. God creates and places us in exactly the time and place needed for us to rise up and accomplish His purpose, if we will accept it. Ephesians 2:10 says, "For we are His handiwork, created in Christ Jesus to do good works, which God prepared in advance for us to do." Hardly any of us will do something as noteworthy as saving an entire peoplehood, but I truly believe we were uniquely designed to overcome the challenges that arise in our lives.

As soon as I heard the voice, I knew that God was essentially telling me, "You are here in this time where there is medicine that can treat you, and you need to take this medicine." And I knew that my outlook had changed. Did I want to go through with it? Absolutely not. But I sighed and accepted my marching orders. I would tell my oncologist of my decision the next day. If God wanted me to do it, there must be a reason, and although I didn't know that reason, the fact that He wanted me to do it was good enough for me. By this time in my life, I trusted Him completely.

One of the foundational experiences that built that trust in God's voice happened back in 2019.

I'm a nurse, and my job involves reviewing notes and applying clinical criteria. This is work that can easily be done from home. Fully remote. But my employer had a hard time accepting that. The company's leadership had a history of flip-flopping on the work-from-home policy every few years, constantly shifting how much remote work was "allowed."

When I was hired, I was told—promised, actually—that after one year, I could transition to 100 percent remote. I didn't get that promise in writing because, up to that point, I had never been double-crossed by an employer. I trusted them.

That turned out to be a huge mistake.

I do not dislike my employer or my line of work. I just had the delusion that corporate America would not change a policy on a whim. I know better now.

Just two months before I hit my one-year anniversary, a new vice president came on board. She had different ideas than our previous VP and department director. She preferred people to be physically present in the office. So, when I asked my supervisor if I could go ahead and go home to work (as I'd been promised), the request went up the chain, was discussed with HR, and came back down as a resounding "no." Not only that, but they started re-evaluating each supervisor's team, looking into who had been allowed to work remotely, and tightening policies across the board.

Our quota is at least twenty cases a day. These can be anything from imaging requests to medical equipment, therapy services, or procedures. Each one has to be carefully reviewed against the most up-to-date, research-based criteria. Then we decide: does it meet the standard, or not?

If it doesn't, we're required to write up a detailed summary for our physician reviewers. A quick, straightforward case might take ten to fifteen minutes. A complicated one could take an hour or more.

Under the new policy, we could technically "earn" the privilege of working from home. But only if we averaged at least thirty cases per day.

I like to think of myself as an optimist. I try to be one. I don't want to be the person always pointing out what's wrong or saying something can't be done. But trust me on this—thirty cases a day? That's impossible if we're doing a full, thorough review like we're supposed to.

Most of us were already pushing ourselves just to hit twenty. Maybe twenty-one on a good day. So, hearing that thirty was now the benchmark to earn back what we had originally been promised? That was crushing.

It wasn't just disappointing. It felt like the rules had changed mid-game.

I was incensed, angry, and bitter. As each day went by, I grew more and more indignant. On top of this, the Army had just given us our moving orders. We were moving; leaving the state. I wanted to keep this job, but I could not do that if they would not let me be remote. I began to feel desperate. The main reason I had taken this job was the promise that I could be remote. Now that promise had been swiftly and utterly revoked and there was nothing I could do about it, as much as I complained.

I was helpless. I pleaded my case to my department supervisor, Erin, that my family was moving due to the military and I did not want to leave this job. I could tell she was disheartened because I had been a good employee and she did not want to lose me, but through our conversation I realized she also felt she could do nothing to help me.

As a last-ditch effort, I reached out to the previous director to beg her for any idea of what I could do, as she had been the one to promise me I could transition to remote work. She responded once to ask if my supervisor had changed but not again after that.

I was powerless. I sat at my desk, spinning my wheels and trying to think of some legal angle to fight the decision—some loophole, some policy, some way to make it right. But I was like grasping at straws.

And even if I *could* find a legal route, did I really want to spend thousands on attorney fees? Drag my employer through the mud? Breed more resentment? Plenty of my coworkers were already fuming, did I want to pour gas on the fire?

I was on the verge of tears when I heard it again. God's voice.

"I will fight *for* you."

The emphasis landed squarely on the *for*. As in, fight in your place. I paused because whenever I perceive the Creator's voice it is awesome enough to give me pause. My soul let out a slow, trembling sigh. I felt my shoulders drop from my ears. I relaxed, albeit only slightly.

I felt some relief, but also confusion. How? How was He going to fight this? What could possibly change in *this* situation? I just did not see what in this world God could do in the circumstances. The VP had said no, she had put out new policies, she had shut this thing down hard. We had to move in three months! I doubted.

I thought, *There's no way. Thanks for the offer, God, but I just don't think it's possible. It's not going to work. I need to just start looking for new jobs. I'll finish this job, but when we move, that's it.* I know I said I'm an optimist but this time it was a bridge too far.

I didn't see a way forward. But apparently, He did.

I decided to look up these words. Just in case they were somewhere in scripture. Like I had with the book of Joshua, I was not certain if these words were anywhere in scripture. Once again, I discovered that they were. And there was a certain parallel to my situation, although mine was far less dire than the one in the Bible. In Exodus 14:13–14, the Israelites were on the run from Pharaoh and his army. Their backs were against the sea, with no way out. Murderous rage glinted in Pharaoh's eye, or so I assume when I play it out in my mind. In fear, the Israelites verbally attack Moses for leading them to their deaths. Moses looks to the Lord and answers them, "Do not be afraid. Stand firm and you will see the deliverance the Lord will bring you today. . . The Lord will fight for you, and you need only be still."

My head was so tired from all the emotions of trying to fight this fight. I desperately needed rest, so I mentally bowed out. *Okay then, God, I will let you fight this instead.* In my heart I did not trust that He would be able to get this done. But I was trying. I was new to hearing and understanding this voice after all, and in my human nature I still thought I would have to do things on my own. I was still trying to see things through earthly eyes.

I gave in. I unclenched my fists, and I laid this knot of fear and frustration in His hands. It was the best I could do.

A month later, as I sat at my desk working, an email popped up on my screen. The subject line caught my eye: "Resignation of VP..."

No way.

I froze, holding my breath. With anticipation, I clicked the email open and began to read.

Sure enough, it said she was moving on to another opportunity and her last day would be a week later. So soon! Erin would make decisions for our department upon the VP's departure. It was too uncanny. Clearly, I could not deny this coincidence. A spark of hope lit up in my heart. Erin had seemed like she wanted me to stay on. Would she now be able to negotiate my remote work with HR? I had no time to waste and I knew I had to ask.

I waited as long as I dared after the VP left. After all, I was on a timeline. If I wanted to keep this job after we moved, an agreement would need to be in place soon. The month of May was nearing its end and our July move date was just around the corner. I went back to Erin and professionally begged again to stay on.

This time, with her additional authority, Erin's face was much less distressed and she smiled and said, "I think this is something we can do. I am going to take it to HR to try to get permission."

God had provided a way within mere weeks. He moved the mountain I had no way of moving. After several more weeks, I had a contract in my hand that said I would get to keep my job and work remotely, permanently. It was more than a contract with my employer. It represented that God saw me, heard me, and answered.

It would have been impossible for me and truthfully, had I pushed more I might have made things worse for myself. He specializes in making a way when there seems to be no way possible. When the Red Sea is in front of us and the enemy is behind. And by the might of man, there is no possible way through. It's only when we stand back and let Him steer that we get to experience the big and small ways that He can provide for us according to His plan. And personally, I think He likes best to do it when we are backed into a corner that seemingly has no way out.

CHAPTER 13

The Tempest

They reeled and staggered like drunkards; they were at their wits'
end. Then they cried out to the Lord in their trouble, and he brought
them out of their distress. He still the storm to a whisper; the waves
of the sea were hushed.

— Psalm 107:27–29 NIV

After the experience where God showed me how He could move the mountains in my life, I trusted Him. I knew God hadn't brought me this far to leave me now.

So, I said yes to the chemotherapy. Yes to trusting that God would once again make a way and get me through it.

As soon as I said yes, the wheels started turning. Fast.

The oncologist wasted no time in setting up my port placement and first infusion. The next step was to have a power port placed in my upper chest. This small device that looks a bit like a soft-edged triangle with two long tails. The surgeon made a small incision near my clavicle and created a pocket under the skin to tuck the port into. From there, he threaded a catheter from the device directly into a vein. Once everything was in place, he closed the skin over the port.

The whole idea is to make chemotherapy easier on your body. Less damage to your veins, fewer IV sticks. I was grateful for that. Anything that could soften the edges of this process, even just a little, felt like a gift.

This surgery went well. And by "well" I mean that I didn't faint. They didn't even put me to sleep. But they did give me a nice dose of something that really relaxed me. There was a lot of pushing and pressure. I remember feeling like the surgeon was putting all of his weight on me. I jokingly said, "Maybe you need to jump on it to get it in?" In my defense, I was pretty loopy from the drugs they gave me. The surgeon, however, didn't seem to appreciate my comedic timing. He gave a deadpan look. Or at least I assume he did because I could not see him. In response he asked the nurse to give me another hit of the relaxant. *Guess my joke didn't land well.*

Because of all the pushing and tugging, the area around my shoulder and up into my neck was sore for about two weeks. The bumps in the car on the way home hurt. There was a large bruise that turned a gross shade of green and then yellow as it faded. To be honest, I hated the port. I could not sleep on my left side the whole time it was in because it was uncomfortable. It was a constant reminder of chemotherapy.

The port left a jagged, thick scar that I will forever call my "Frankenstein scar." It wasn't the first scar I'd earned that year, and it wouldn't be the last. The scars from the surgery on my right side (to remove the tumor and test my lymph nodes) were nice, thin, clean cuts that were fading to a faint white color. They were already fading into faint white traces, barely noticeable now. But they stood in stark contrast to the angry, red, H-shaped mark on my left side. What all the scars had in common, though, was that each of them left behind sensitive tissue. They were small, physical reminders of the battle waged underneath.

I winced as I bent over to pick up the backpack I was packing for infusion day. The port site was still exquisitely painful. It hurt to look up or down or bend over. It was an unsightly large lump under my skin in triangular form with three small bumps sticking up. The other part of it that I could feel was up either under or over my collarbone; I'm still not sure which. I never got over the feeling of a hard piece of plastic up by my neck for the year that I would have that foreigner in my body.

There was no time wasted between inserting the port and starting chemotherapy. For me it was three days, but one of the oncology infusion nurses told me that some people begin their treatments the very same day the port goes in. I was thankful they hadn't tried to access mine right away.

When it was time, I put my blue backpack on the bed. It had once belonged to my son, in kindergarten. He'd outgrown it now, needing a bigger one for books and his school-issued laptop. I've never liked throwing useful things away, so it had been sitting in his closet until I remembered I'd need to bring a lot of supplies on infusion days. It felt like the right choice; something small and familiar, a piece of home to carry with me into the unknown.

I packed a soft blanket, ear pods, a magazine, my new glasses (which I now needed thanks to the aging process), snacks, an external charger for my phone, and my new book.

Knowing I would be spending up to six hours each infusion day at the cancer center, I decided I needed something encouraging to help pass the time. I went onto a Christian distributor website and looked for something to spark my interest. Wouldn't you know it—less than two weeks after I heard God whisper to me through Esther, the first thing I saw was a book titled *You Were Made for This Moment* by Max Lucado. It is based on the book of Esther. I instantly knew that I needed to get that book. Small coincidences.

The snacks that I packed were lovingly supplied by a whole community of people. When I agreed to do chemotherapy, I was not sure how I would feel or how nauseous I would be. Not knowing what else to do, I took to Facebook and created a wish list on Amazon of various things to try that might be okay for my tummy. So many people were reaching out and asking me what they could do and I had trouble thinking of anything for them to do. I was blessed to not have any expenses, although a lot of people going through cancer treatment have bills stacked high, so a GoFundMe did not seem necessary. I thought a wish list might be a good way for people to give to me if they really wanted to.

I added anything I could think of to the list, expecting maybe 10 percent of it would actually get purchased. But the moment I posted it on my Facebook page, friends and family flocked to Amazon and started buying. Within two hours, not a single item remained. Some things even had duplicates. I was shocked. Overwhelmed. People had shown up for me when I needed them most. We really are better in a community than we are alone. If only they all could have come with me for the infusions…

I sighed. Packing helped because at least I was doing something. Whenever I sat still, the nerves crept in. Questions started swirling. How would chemo make me feel? Would I throw up? I detested throwing up. Would it work? Would I lose my hair? Would I be able to keep my job?

The tempest was starting again, threatening to take me away. I was learning that life can easily become a tornado and pick you up with it if you're not anchored to something. The only thing I know of that's strong enough to withstand the storms of life is Jesus (see Matthew 8:23–27). I didn't know it but the storm was about to become a full-blown gale.

CHAPTER 14

The Sparrow and the Hawk

"Look at the birds of the air; they do not sow or reap or store away in barns, and yet your heavenly Father feeds them. Are you not much more valuable than they? Can any one of you by worrying add a single hour to your life?"

— Matthew 6:26 NIV

I was a bundle of nerves as I drove to the cancer center for my first infusion. My port site was still tender, covered with a bandage, and every movement reminded me it was there. I tried to gather my courage as I walked through the entrance, past the smiling faces at the front desk who waved me in like I was a regular. I made my way to the bright common room with its own separate greeting desk. The space was dressed in hues of brown, gray, and off-white—calm, neutral colors, maybe chosen to soothe.

The pleasant ladies at the desk took my name, printed labels, and told me I could sit wherever I liked. The room had a wall of windows that opened to a small courtyard, a TV mounted on the far wall, and a collection of wide chairs arranged in a semicircle. I chose one right by the window so I could look out at the trees and sky. I was the first patient there. It wasn't even 8 a.m.

The first order of business was to draw my blood and make sure everything looked okay to start the infusion. The nurse asked if I wanted lidocaine. I looked at the needle she was holding. It was the biggest needle I had ever seen—roughly the size of a lapel pin. "Yes, please!"

She peeled off the bandage, which I'd been instructed not to remove myself. Underneath, the site still had dried, caked flecks of blood and an angry purple bruise. She grabbed a small aerosol can and began spraying the absolute coldest spray I have ever felt. I was shocked! It actually burned. I had expected a quick spritz, but she kept going. The cold became sharp, almost like a shot. I winced.

Once she finished, she asked me to sit all the way back against the backrest and brace myself. I tilted my head back and lowered my shirt to try to give her as much access to this thing as possible. Piercing pain went through me as she pushed the huge needle through my skin and into my port. But once over, I finally sat back and relaxed a little.

I had wondered how an infusion could take all day, and I certainly found out that first day. After my bloodwork was drawn, the needle stayed in my port with tubing left attached for the upcoming infusion—so they didn't have to stick me twice. I was *very* grateful for that. It had hurt badly enough *with* the numbing spray. I couldn't imagine the pain without it.

Then I had to meet with the pharmacist. I had an entire batch of new medications. It is truly amazing how many medications are prescribed to a cancer patient to combat the side effects of chemotherapy: Three different drugs for nausea alone. Another for diarrhea. Another to help with bone pain. Another to decrease adverse reactions and inflammation brought on by the chemo itself.

If this wasn't enough, you don't just take the medications when you have the pain or nausea, some of them are on a specific schedule. Take this med twice a day on the day before, day of, and day after your infusion. Take this med once a day for seven days leading up to your infusion. Take this med at bedtime for the first four days following your infusion. Take the rest as needed, but not too often, and call us if you need to take them. Holy moly! Luckily, they take into account how overwhelming this can be and give you a nice printed schedule of when to take everything.

Once I was done with the pharmacist, it was time to see the oncologist. We would meet every infusion day to talk about side effects and to see how my labs were doing. I was scheduled for a dose-dense schedule of every two weeks. This chemotherapy drug is lovingly referred to as "The Red Devil" because of its appearance. It gets its nickname from its vivid, Kool-Aid–red color. Also because of the brutal reputation it carries.

The nurse had to be decked out in full hazmat gear and take special precautions just to administer it. She didn't even touch the actual liquid. That made me wince a little because if she needed layers of protection just to handle the stuff, and couldn't even come into direct contact with it, how was it safe to pump it straight into my body? Right into my heart. But my bloodwork came back fine, and since it was my first infusion, everything was a go. Which meant—it was time for the drugs.

In between all of these activities, I sat in my comfy chair and stared out the window. I couldn't believe I was here, doing this, at the age of thirty-nine. Life had really thrown me for a loop with this one. And yet, I couldn't help but count my blessings in the midst of the chaos. If I had not found the lump when I did, it could have been stage 3 or even 4 (metastatic cancer, which is incurable). And I reminded myself: I had been healthy my entire life until now. There are people who fight much worse battles than I would have to. That perspective helped me breathe through the fear.

My thoughts also turned toward my family. I had a loving and supportive partner in this fight. I had a good job. We had good insurance, even though this Tricare provider had frustrated me in the beginning of my journey. What does a single mother do? What if she doesn't have insurance or has terrible insurance? What if she barely makes ends meet in her job and now is faced with having to take a ton of time off for appointments and treatment? What would I do in her shoes? It's tempting to ignore your health and keep working for your kids. But if the cancer progresses and your kids don't have you around, they are in worse shape. So what do you do?

I had a lot of time to think. Some people dread being alone with their thoughts, but I welcome the quiet. It's the only time I feel like I can sort through the noise in my head. I looked out the large windows. Outside the window, a nature documentary was playing out in real time. A small sparrow sat motionless on the concrete walkway. It looked injured, dazed. I kept glancing back at it, and for hours it didn't move.

Then I noticed a hawk perched in a nearby tree. It had spotted the little bird, too. Surely, I thought, something cataclysmic was about to happen. I watched intently, bracing for the moment the hawk would swoop down, talons outstretched, and snatch the helpless sparrow. It wasn't looking good for the sparrow, who seemed barely conscious.

As I alternated watching outside and reading, the nurse came and went, hooking up one IV, disconnecting another. Unfortunately, you don't just get to start chemotherapy and then leave once it's finished. First, they give you fluids. Those have to go in over an hour. After that you have to wait a half hour. Then it's a steroid. That one is a little faster and only takes about twenty minutes. But after that one you have to wait almost an hour. Then comes a type of medication that is like an antacid. This is very necessary as sour stomach or acid reflux pain would become a bane as my treatments continued. There is another wait after that one is infused, to let it take effect. Finally, you can get to the actual chemotherapy, about four or five hours after first sitting in the chair. By the time the nurse connected the chemotherapy I felt like I had already run a marathon just sitting still.

The type of chemotherapy used for my breast cancer is actually two drugs, given one after the other. They examine the cancer cells under a microscope to determine the specific type, and each kind has its own treatment. Before administering it, the nurse has to put on a plastic apron, special gloves, and a face shield. Then another nurse has to sign off on my chart to confirm I'm receiving the correct medication in the right amount. I, on the other hand, have no protection from this toxic drug and am about to receive it directly into my veins. It was surreal—the contrast between all the precautions they took and my complete exposure. I suddenly didn't want to watch what was unfolding in front of me. I turned my gaze back outside.

To my surprise, the small sparrow appeared to be much better. She had brightened up and no longer looked like she was on the brink of death. The hawk was gone. She began hopping around and, within minutes, flew away. I felt like cheering right in the middle of the infusion center. As I watched her go, it dawned on me—there's a scripture passage about sparrows. See Luke 12:6–7: "Yet not one sparrow is forgotten by God. Even the hairs of your head have all been counted. So do not be afraid; you are worth much more than many sparrows!"

Overall, sparrows in the Bible represent God's love and care for His creation, as well as the importance of humility and trust in God's provision. God was again using small signs to communicate with me. Small coincidences. In that moment, I realized:

I was the sparrow. Weakened, vulnerable, exposed to danger I couldn't fight on my own. And cancer—that looming shadow over my life—was the hawk. But just like the sparrow, I wasn't forgotten. I wasn't alone. God had seen me, protected me, and reminded me, even through a small bird and a window, that He was near.

CHAPTER 15

"I Want to Quit"

For our light and momentary troubles are achieving for us an eternal glory that far outweighs them all. So we fix our eyes not on what is seen, but what is unseen, since what is seen is temporary, but what is unseen is eternal.

— 2 Corinthians 4:17–18 NIV

I walked out of the infusion center six hours after I arrived. It was cool outside. The world was still very much in the grips of winter; typical of mid-February. I drove home, feeling tired but fine and hoping that would continue so I could work for two hours like I had planned to do. Once I got home and logged on to my computer, I started feeling a little fluish. It was mild at first (some joint pain and a creeping fatigue), but it steadily got worse as the day went on. Still, I pushed through and managed to finish working. By the time I wrapped up, though, the sick feeling had settled in deeper, and I was more than ready to be done for the day.

It was a low-key evening and I went to bed early. I was unsure what the next few days would bring as far as symptoms and I was nervous about how bad it might be. But I knew I had the medications they had given me so I had hopes that it wouldn't be too bad. I looked at each bottle before going to bed, checking it against my calendar the pharmacist had given me. I took the pills I was supposed to take. I made some space in my nightstand drawer and put all the pills in there. I said my prayers and turned out the light. Bill reached for my hand in the darkness.

I awoke sometime before dawn and immediately felt off. Intense nausea greeted me and a new type of feeling. It was like weakness and exhaustion and an odd sensation in the bottom of my throat. Thinking I would throw up soon, I made my way to the bathroom and assumed the universal gastric distress position. My breath was coming fast and shallow. I broke out in a cold sweat. The world was fading and my last thought was, *Wait, I know what this is, this is not puking, this is fainting*, and then all went dark.

I was not out long, mere seconds likely. I was now on our bath mat, staring up at the ceiling. I was thankful we had gotten such a soft, padded bath mat now. My feet were on the cold floor. I felt so awful. There was no way I would be able to get up, I could feel already that it would not be possible anytime soon. I called out for my husband. I hated waking him but I was incapacitated at the moment. No response. *Crap*. I tried again, louder. Bill came wandering into the bathroom rubbing his eyes and half asleep. "Are you okay?" he asked.

"Can you get my pills?" That was all I could manage to get out. I meant my anti-nausea pills, but I could not say this. I was still incredibly nauseous and afraid that if I were to say more, then I would start throwing up. Bill left and after he was gone I realized he probably had no idea my pills were in my nightstand, and on top of that he wouldn't know which ones to bring out of the seven or so bottles.

He returned, still looking bleary-eyed, with his arms wrapped around two pillows. I couldn't help but laugh out loud. Despite how awful I felt, I was grateful I still had a sense of humor. "Not pillows, pills!" I still smile every time I think back on that moment. God bless my sweet husband and his ever-helping heart.

I would spend the next several days sleeping twelve hours or more each night, taking my anti-nausea medications whenever I was allowed to, and feeling horrible. I was still nauseous despite maxing out the medications. I had a small device on my arm with a needle embedded in my skin. It was programmed to inject medicine two days after my infusion.

Because this type of chemotherapy can make your white blood cells drop low enough to be concerning, doctors give an injection that stimulates your body to make these cells. Sure enough, when it was supposed to do its thing, I heard a series of clicks and then a small whirring noise. "I'm getting my medicine!" I announced to Bill.

Twenty-four hours later, I was hurting on an unimaginable level. I was warned that the stimulating drug, called Neulasta, causes bone pain. But I was on medication to help prevent this pain. An allergy medication of all things, taken for seven days surrounding the injection, is a wonder drug for the bone pain from Neulasta—supposedly. This is what my medical team wanted me to believe.

Instead, I don't think it did anything for me. It may as well have been a placebo. I sat on the couch in the worst pain I had been in since my non-medicated labor with my son. Tears were now spilling silently down my cheeks as I sat on the couch, so I knew the pain was about the same as early labor. Now I sat with my bones feeling like each one had been hit with a baseball bat. Sitting was excruciating on my back. I couldn't have my children hug me because it hurt. I couldn't have my husband massage my muscles because they too were sore. I could feel my clothes on my skin, and even that somehow made my bones ache.

I was beyond miserable, completely exhausted. All I wanted was for the pain to stop. It hurt so badly. And there was no escape. No way to make it go away.

I turned to Bill. "I can't stay awake any more, I'm going to bed." I was hoping the pain would be gone by the time I woke up.

Bill got up and came to me. He gently helped me get up. He wrapped his arm around me and supported me. We meandered slowly, step-by-step down the hall toward the bedroom. Although it physically hurt to have him prop me up, emotionally it was exactly what I needed. The nausea and pain from the first round of chemotherapy were more than I could take. *There's no way I can do this five more times.* I messaged my doctor: "I want to quit."

She immediately got back to me through the portal, wanting to set up a visit to discuss it with me ASAP. Thankfully, Dr. Dowell did not try to shame me or bully me into any certain decision, although I'm sure she had a preference. She laid out the options like a professional. We could stay the course and add some more supportive medications, or there was research that supported switching to a different regimen. The alternate regimen did have about a 1 percent drop in efficiency long-term. Instead of a dose every two weeks, this treatment would be once every three weeks. That change would eliminate the need for the dreaded Neulasta shot that made all my bones feel broken. This other treatment also had a reputation for having more manageable side effects.

To me, the choice seemed clear. "Let's switch!" I now had four treatments ahead of me, and with that, a new question began to loom over me was whether I would lose my hair. he thought of it filled me with dread, and I had a sinking feeling I would. Every woman I knew who had gone through chemotherapy for breast cancer had lost her hair. ill, however, remained optimistic, reassuring me several times, "You may not lose it." I hoped he was right, but I prepared for the worst.

I bought several wigs, head coverings, and hats that I liked. I am eternally grateful for Amazon and the ability to buy anything there that you can possibly think of. I didn't try them on to see how they looked and if I liked them. I figured if my hair fell out, how they looked wouldn't matter because I wouldn't have a choice. I might look silly in the covers I bought, but I'd look sillier as a bald woman.

About two weeks after my first treatment, my scalp became fiercely tender. Sure enough, within the next day my hair started to fall out. You might wonder how one can tell when their hair is falling out in this way, because we all experience hair shedding in the shower or in the hairbrush and sometimes think, "Wow, that's a lot of hair." But this is different. The hair comes out in clumps, as though there is no root attached—and, I suppose, there probably isn't.

Chemotherapy changes all of your skin, any cell that grows quickly. The aim is to disrupt that process so that cancer cells can't multiply. But it's not a specific process. It is indiscriminate. Any cell that is trying to reproduce is harmed. Thus, you get an array of symptoms depending on the type of skin affected.

The inside of your mouth develops sores. Your taste buds go haywire. I could hardly taste most food and the ones that I could taste were nothing like how I remembered them nor what they should be. It was highly unsatisfying. I would crave carbs, like a heaping plate of cheesy potatoes. I would make said potatoes, and then be completely disappointed when I took a bite as it tasted like cardboard to me. And yes, it also makes your hair fall out.

I tried to brush my hair, but copious amounts of it were left in the brush. I decided not to brush any more of it. It was time to make the decision I had been dreading since the start of all this. As luck would have it, I already had an appointment with my hair stylist in a few days. It was an appointment that I had made six months prior, before I even knew that I had cancer.

I went online and started researching organizations that take hair donations. Each had slightly different rules on the minimum length they would take and whether the hair could be dyed. I even checked reviews and where much of their profits went. I decided on Wigs for Kids because I was not sure I could make the minimum length requirement of some of the others. Plus, they specialize in children with hair loss. Who could turn their back on a child?

It's not that I had amazing, beautiful hair that I styled regularly—I definitely didn't. My hair was often a bit messy and quite frizzy. I frequently lamented that I couldn't stand it. Most days, I just threw it into a ponytail so I wouldn't have to deal with it. But it was mine, and sometimes, I suppose, it could even be pretty. It was coffee brown (with a few grays creeping in at the top) and wavy. If I wanted to get fancy, I'd put some mousse in while it was wet and let it air dry to curls—that was the extent of my styling.

Still, being a woman, there's just something about your hair that feels deeply personal. It defines you, at least in part. It represents a piece of your femininity. It's one of the first things people notice about you. I knew it was illogical to get so worked up about losing my hair—after all, how important is hair in the grand scheme of things? But that realization didn't make me feel any better about losing it.

CHAPTER 16

Crowning Glory

The Lord is close to the brokenhearted and saves those who are crushed in spirit.

— Psalm 34:18 NIV

The day that I was to shave my head, Bill took the kids to run errands with him so I could have the day to myself. I picked out a head wrap from my drawer. I caught sight of my Bible and opened it. I read 1 Corinthians 11:15: "But if a woman has long hair, it is a glory to her; for her hair is given to her for a covering." Then I cried. I was so scared. I dreaded what needed to be done. I considered canceling the appointment and just letting it fall out one long piece after another.

But I couldn't do that. I wanted someone to be able to use my hair. And if it wasn't going to be me, then I would send it to another. I dried my tears as best I could and tried not to think about my current situation, because every time I did the tears came afresh. I got in the car and headed to my salon.

Brenda, my usual stylist, was waiting for me. I explained what was going on and why I wanted to shave my head. I asked her to save the hair because I was going to donate it. She nodded solemnly and after a wash we began. She put my hair in three ponytails. The last ponytails I would have for who knows how long, I pondered. Brenda extended the clippers and asked if I wanted to make the first cut.

No way, I can't be the one to make myself ugly, I thought. But all I said was a soft, "No." She started buzzing. The ponytails came off quickly. Buzz, buzz, buzz. Then she just had to even it up. My scalp was hurting but there was nothing that could be done about it. I stared in silent horror as I watched my head transform into something I hated the look of. I started crying all over again. I couldn't help it.

Brenda calmly stopped buzzing. She fished out a tissue and handed it to me, then said, "Your hair is not your crowning glory. Your personality is, and you're beautiful inside and out."

If there had been a record playing, I'm convinced it would have come to a scratching stop. What on earth?! I was utterly baffled. Her exact choice of words; how did she know precisely what I had read just a couple hours before?

But I also knew that these coincidences are just too ... coincidental to be happenstance. I knew, and still know, that it was God. Whispering to me through another human soul that He was there with me, still loved me, felt the pain of losing my hair with me. It was like a Band-aid for my soul, albeit temporary. Small coincidences.

When all the hair was off, I put on a purple head cover and collected my hair in a bag. Then I came home and stared at myself in the mirror. My face was bloated and puffy from all of the chemotherapy fluids. My eyes were red and swollen from crying. I looked old. Tired. I looked like Gollum. (I didn't even think I was that big of a *Lord of the Rings* fan, but here I am—two references deep.)

I did not like what I saw, so I stopped looking. It would take six months before I could look at my head again with anything other than repulsion. Six months before I had anything more than stubble on my head. And six months before I would look in the mirror and like my reflection again. I got in the shower to wash the stray hairs off. In the shower, I cried some more—harder this time, as I watched what was left of my hair slowly swirl down the drain.

But then, in the quiet of the shower, God's voice whispered another Bible verse to my heart. It was Luke 12:7: "Indeed, the very hairs of your head are all numbered." (NIV) Once again I was soothed. I knew that if God knew exactly how many hairs I had, then He truly cared for me. He didn't want me to lose my hair any more than I did.

Can you imagine loving someone enough to count how many hairs are on their head? I knew that God gives beauty for ashes. I knew He would faithfully turn things around. If not in this life, certainly in the next.

Feeling slightly better, I packed the three thirteen-inch-long ponytails of hair in a padded mail sleeve. (I know the length because I had to measure them to make sure they were long enough for donation). I made plans to mail the package the next day. I found it comforting to imagine a small child receiving a beautiful wig for her small head with patchy or no hair of her own. If I couldn't use my hair anymore, someone should be able to benefit from it, doggone it.

Many months later, I would also Google "hair as a crowning glory." I found a website that sums up my metamorphosis exactly at this stage. It says, "apart from adorning it in various styles, the deeper significance of hair is undeniable. It is the extension of our opinions, beliefs and who we are becoming. Similar to our mental and physical wellness, hair is deeply connected to our emotional health and spiritual identity."[1]

I couldn't believe how it paralleled scripture. I was physically becoming a new creation, starting over from scratch. 2 Corinthians 5:17 says, "Therefore, if anyone is in Christ, the new creation has come. The old has gone, the new is here!" (NIV) I could literally see the outward representation of the inward work God was doing in me. And I knew someday He would give me beauty for ashes (see Isaiah 61:3).

---

1 Nombuso Kumalo and Nomvelo Masango, "Sacred Threads: The Spiritual Significance of Hair," *SowetanLIVE*, June 7, 2021, https://www.sowetanlive.co.za/good-life/2021-06-07-sacred-threads-the-spiritual-significance-of-hair/.

CHAPTER 17

Toughing It Out

"I will refresh the weary and satisfy the faint."
— Jeremiah 31:25 NIV

Losing my hair felt like losing a layer of protection, a part of my identity that let me blend in. Now, every time I looked in the mirror, I barely recognized the woman staring back. But the hardest part wasn't what I saw; it was what everyone else would see.

I have always been quiet. I prefer to be as inconspicuous as a fly on the wall. I do not like attention. Having a bald head felt like a curse to me. It drew everyone's attention as much as if I were strolling around naked. Thomas and Grace were in baseball and softball that spring. I would don a head wrap and venture to the ball fields. I tried to tiptoe in with my camping chair. *Nothing to see here. Please don't stare at me.*

But people did stare. I suppose they didn't know what to make of a young-ish woman with no hair. My least favorite part was "the look." If my eyes met theirs, they'd give me that expression—one of pity. I don't want to seem ungrateful. I truly appreciate that they felt sympathy. But it was also a painful reminder that my struggle was visible. There was no hiding it. No way to keep my treatment private or to take a break from it—not even for an hour at the ball field to watch my kids swing a bat. Their pity reminded me that, to the outside world, I was pitiable.

It was during my chemotherapy that my mom began to form a plan to have her treatment closer to family. She lived many states away from my brother and me, and she was worried that with a strict therapy regimen she would miss out on the entire summer with her four grandchildren. I took action and called my oncologist's office. I asked whether my mom could come to them. The girl at the front desk assured me that as long as my mom got a referral, she would be allowed. My mom got her referral and with that we set in motion a scheme to have my mom complete her treatment at the exact same facility where I was getting mine.

Although our infusion days were never the same, it was somehow comforting to have my mom going through the same awful journey, and at the same place and time. We got to know all the "girls" (nurses) at our infusion center and took pleasure in conversing with them during our visits. My mom was quickly versed in the local gossip from car accidents to the goings-on behind the scenes of the county fair. We had our preferred chairs and our routines. The staff was nearly giddy to be simultaneously treating a mother/daughter combo at the same time. They said it was the first time it had happened. Every time I went in for an infusion, the girls had to tell me how sweet and wonderful my mom was. Of course, I already knew this, she's my mom!

The next few months while I completed my chemotherapy were a blur of exhaustion, nausea, constipation, then diarrhea (oh yes, you get two for the price of one with chemo), a cyclic rash on my face every week after an infusion, and everything tasting awful. It's kind of like signing up for a gastrointestinal bug every three weeks. In other words, I hated it.

I wore headscarves for the most part rather than wigs. I thought the wigs looked too fake, and when I wore them, they were itchy and painful on my sensitized head. I wanted to wear them and feign normalcy for strangers even if I knew the reality. But it was just too uncomfortable.

I went to visit my primary care doctor in the midst of chemotherapy. During the intake process, her nurse went through the typical depression questionnaire. Not surprisingly, I didn't score very well. I was starting to feel hopeless again—the familiar sensation of heavy weights shackled to my ankles, slowly dragging me down.

I hadn't been able to walk much during treatment, so exercise was out of the question. And since everything tasted awful, I wasn't eating healthy. Carbs were the only thing that didn't have a metallic, battery-acid taste. I felt so crummy most of the time that I couldn't even bring myself to take vitamins. Thinking positively felt impossible.

I don't know if chemotherapy messes with your brain chemistry, but it wouldn't surprise me. It certainly felt like it did. One by one, all of my usual strategies to keep the beast of depression at bay were failing.

I waited for my doctor to come into the exam room, really hoping she would ask me about my answers to the questionnaire. Dr. Carson came in with her wonderful, cheerful smile. Well, her eyes smiled a lot. Her actual smile was hidden behind a mask and I had never seen it. She is a great doctor and from the first time I had an appointment with her I immediately felt at ease. That is not the case with most doctors as far as I'm concerned. After some small talk and asking me about a few aches and pains and how treatment was going, she brought it up.

"So, you've got some depression going on, huh?"

I couldn't hold back the tears. Like a cracked dam held together with Scotch tape, they were constantly at the ready lately. The slightest acknowledgment from another human about how difficult this had all been was enough to break it wide open. I told her how low I really felt. How I'd had a passive death wish in the past and felt I was getting close to that once more. She looked at me with deep sympathy and gently asked, "Is it alright if I give you a hug?"

That was the first—and only—time a doctor has ever hugged me. I can't fully express how meaningful it was in that moment. I will forever be grateful to her for that. As she wrapped her arms around me, she spoke words that went straight to my soul.

"It's okay for you to feel crappy, because cancer is being very mean to you and it's not fair."

Her honesty brought a ghost of a smile to my lips.

She agreed to refer me for cognitive behavioral therapy, which I completed over the next two months. I did feel it helped, though it was tough to juggle alongside the physical toll of treatment and the demands of work. There were so many symptoms to manage—on top of the depression that was still creeping in, its icy fingers reaching for my soul. Even so, I was committed to continuing work throughout treatment, mostly because I couldn't afford to lose my job.

One day in particular was quite rough. I felt off from the moment I woke up. My head seemed to be spinning. The world moved from right to left in a blur, then sailed back and started over. Nothing would stand still. The longer I sat up, the worse I felt. I did not want to take the day off; I had precious little time off left after all the doctor's appointments and infusions. I sat at my desk, nauseous, dizzy, and miserable. It was slightly better I found if I put my head down. But not a lot.

Obviously, I couldn't work without looking at my computer and typing. I tried in vain to raise my head and work in small bits, only to have the awful feeling return. My body was so tired. I just wanted to lie down. Maybe for just a minute . . .

I tried it. It felt much better. The nausea abated; the dizziness subsided. I ended up spending the afternoon working in spurts as fast as I could followed by sessions of lying down under my desk. Thank goodness I did not have to be in an office. Only with the help of God did I meet my productivity goal that day.

Time during chemo seemed to crawl at a snail's pace. It was divided into three stages: the days leading up to an infusion, when I had to make sure to take all my preloading meds; infusion day, when I was pumped full of enough fluid to quench the thirst of a small village and gained at least five pounds with every treatment; and then the aftermath.

By that point, my nail beds were sore, with red streaks across my nails. Worst of all, my nails were starting to separate from my fingers. When I looked at them head-on, I could see a gap between each nail and the finger it was supposed to be attached to. But with the last infusion day approaching, my anticipation was building. I wouldn't say I was excited, but there was certainly a sense of levity. A weight was being lifted from me, and I was just glad to get it over with.

Bill asked if he could come and watch me ring the bell after my last round. I was honored that he would want to come. So many people are squeamish when it comes to cancer. They don't know what to say, so they don't talk to you. They are uncomfortable with your appearance, so they don't come around. And I don't blame them at all. Before I was drawn into the whirlwind of cancer, I felt awkward around those with it also. The blessing of having my husband by my side, supporting me without hesitation, was something I deeply appreciated.

After my final infusion, the nurses and some of the front desk staff gathered near the bell. Out of nowhere, a sweet older lady appeared, radiating happy support, a moment I still cherish. Bill was there too, capturing it all on video for me. With all the strength I could muster, I rang that bell as hard as I could.

The next order of business in my treatment plan was radiation. This was not daunting to me. My mom had breezed through it so I figured I would too. Plus, after the trauma that had been chemotherapy, I figured there was no way that radiation could be worse. Fortunately, it wasn't.

Because of my age and the aggressive nature of my cancer, the radiation oncologist recommended thirty-two rounds of radiation to target an entire quadrant, which included all of the surrounding lymph nodes. This decision was based on the fact that cancer had been found in two out of the four lymph nodes that were sampled. As a result, the radiation treatment covered an area from my neck, around to my back, to the midline, and down to my ribs.

There were only two downsides. The first was that my arms would go numb every time. The radiation for each type of cancer has to be treated in a different position. And since each person's body is different, they have to create a mold of each person. In order to do this, you have to hold absolutely still for about an hour as they contort your body in a form of origami torture.

Holding my arms above my head for anywhere from twenty to forty-five minutes each session left my hands numb and tingly and my shoulders ached ferociously. So many times I would think in my head, *I can't do it this time. I have to move, I HAVE to bring my arms down just for a second, just a little relief.*

But then I would remember some of my breathing techniques. I had to do the breathing techniques slowly and carefully so I would not move my body too much and risk messing up the very precise points they drew on my skin where the exacting beam of radiation had to be aligned perfectly for every pass. Deep breath in. Hold the breath. Clear my mind. Focus on the breath. Slowly exhale, slowly, slowly. It got me through the pain and numbness.

The other challenge was the burn from the radiation. Through a strict regimen of heavy lotion, concentrated green tea spray, prescription-strength lidocaine, and ice—along with the oversight of my radiation oncologist—I was able to protect most of my skin.

But there was a small rectangular patch just above my clavicle that developed an intense, angry, red burn. No matter what I tried, it just got worse and more painful. It was itchy and hot, and it hurt. The skin felt raw, inflamed, and blistered. It burned like a sunburn, but far more viciously.

I only had a few days left, but I was tempted to skip them, to give my skin a much-needed break. Yet, quitting was never an option for me. So, I pushed through the pain and finished the radiation treatments like a champ. Despite the agony, my skin stayed intact, though it felt like I had dragged it across a searing-hot sharpening stone. But, thank God, it didn't open up. The final day came and went quietly, and just like that, I was done with all my active cancer treatments. My battle with cancer was over. But God was not done with me.

CHAPTER 18

Steadfast Anchor

Look to the Lord and his strength, seek his face always.
— 1 Chronicles 16:11 NIV

October is Breast Cancer Awareness Month. Coincidentally, it is also my birth month and the month I was diagnosed with breast cancer. I wish I could just be "aware" of breast cancer on the sidelines, a spectator if you will. But I was pulled into this fight long before I should have been, and this monster doesn't fight fair. Because I have a genetic mutation that reduces my body's ability to repair damaged DNA, I am more likely to get certain cancers. And the odds can be scary. I had up to a 60 percent chance of developing breast cancer in my life (check that box). I still have at least a 25 percent chance of developing a second breast cancer at some point. I have up to a 30 percent risk of developing ovarian cancer (by comparison, the average woman's risk is 1 percent). And my risk of pancreatic cancer is somewhere between 5 and 10 percent, again the average person's risk is 1 percent.

What do you do with the knowledge of these statistics? Once you know them, you can't forget. How do you go about living a semblance of a normal life with these thoughts at the back of your mind? My ordeal with depression taught me that if I look for joy in this world, I know I will not find it there. The only joy that I have found is in the hope that comes through Jesus. I cling to that when faced with travails.

I decided on risk-reducing surgery after careful consideration of the statistics. The surgery is a total hysterectomy and removal of both ovaries. It was set for October—Breast Cancer Awareness Month and one year after I found out I had breast cancer. Once again, I was asked to fast. This time for forty-eight hours.

The first day was the same as a colonoscopy prep. Clear liquid and lots of Miralax. The second day was water only. I had started doing an occasional fast with prayer to grow spiritually. Only for one meal here and there. It made me nervous because of my past experiences with fainting anytime I skipped a meal. The more I practiced fasting, the easier it became. It is also a great practice for relying on God and drawing closer to Him since each time you feel a hunger pang you thank God for what you do have and pray for help with completing the fast. Perhaps one of the best benefits is that it helped change my relationship with food. I realized I had started to use food to bring comfort, and I was way too into requiring a sweet treat to feel satisfied for the day.

Fasting once in a while made me see food as nourishment rather than an entitlement.

But when fasting for medical reasons, it takes you to a whole different headspace. By the second night of this fast I was hungry, tired, probably irritable, and ready to call it a night early just to put myself out of misery. I wanted the day of surgery to come (and go) faster so I could get back to eating. I woke up in the middle of the night to go to the bathroom. As soon as I stood up, I felt funny.

Once in the bathroom, trouble hit. My breathing rate quickened. I had a sense of dread. I broke out in a cold sweat. Now hyperventilating and weak, my head slowly slumped to the side until it was resting on the countertop. The last thing I remember was staring at the light.

When I came back around, I realized I had fainted, again. I was only out for a moment. This was becoming too much of a routine surrounding medical procedures. I could barely stand because I was so weak from not eating for two days. I went back to bed slowly, carefully, expecting my legs to give out at any moment. Afraid my blood sugar was low, I took a sip of Gatorade even though I was only supposed to be having water at this point. Bill woke up and I told him I had fainted. I began shivering uncontrollably. He took me in his arms and in a matter of minutes I warmed up and fell asleep, my ordeal nearly forgotten.

When we got to the surgery center the next day and got checked in, everything was going smoothly until they gave me the pre-surgery drug cocktail. I can't say I remember all of the drugs but it was some mix of Oxycodone, Tylenol, Dilaudid, and probably a few others I am forgetting. These are to be given about a half hour prior to surgery in order to lessen the pain after the operation.

The problem came just after they gave me the pharmaceutical cocktail, when we learned that my surgery would be delayed because the case ahead of mine was taking a long time.

Right around the time that I should have been wheeled back to the operating room, I began feeling nauseous. Really nauseous. Of course a nurse is never available at the drop of a hat, so by the time Bill found mine I was dry heaving into a plastic puke holder. The nurse sprang into action and got some anti-nausea medicine to give me through my IV and a bag of fluids.

That is about the last thing I remember except for bits and pieces of eating and walking after my surgery. I did stay one night as they wanted me to. Bill picked me up the next day. But largely, I don't recall. Anesthesia is a funny thing. Large chunks are missing from my memory after this surgery for at least twenty-four hours afterward. I am pretty sure my parents came to help with my kids but I was so out of it that I'm not even sure of this simple fact.

The recovery after this surgery was fairly low-key. At least this surgery went better than the procedure to remove the chemotherapy port. That takes the cake for my all-time least favorite procedure ever. Had I known that they were not going to use any anesthesia, not even a tiny bit, and just a little slather of lidocaine, I would have refused the procedure. My skin was not completely numb when they cut into me and I could slightly feel the blade slicing through. I looked for my nurse.

"I'm getting very nauseous," I told her.

She scrambled for the anti-nausea medication. She nervously read my blood pressure to the surgeon: "72/40." I could tell she was not happy to see me tanking like this as she hooked up a bolus (fluids to boost your blood pressure).

"Vasovagal," the surgeon calmly replied. That just means that someone is fainting because of stress.

Had they known that my brain would initiate a shutdown sequence and they would need interventions, they probably would have given me that anesthesia. When they wheeled me back into my room, Bill was waiting for me. I couldn't form words to convey the amount of discomfort I had just gone through, another fainting spell, and the icky factor of feeling a scalpel cut into my skin.

"That sucked," was all I could manage.

* * *

I began counting the cost of what I had been through in the last year. I now had eight new scars on my torso. I had lost my hair. I was weak. I felt sick. After the surgeries my weight kept dropping even though I was not trying. At one hundred and seven pounds, I now felt frail (no need to worry, I have since gained it all back and then some). I was not seeing myself in a positive light when I looked in the mirror.

But through it all, my husband was my steadfast anchor. When I talked about how much I hated my short hair, he would insist it was cute. When I moaned about my new scars, he would say he liked them because they marked that I was still here — I hadn't passed away.

Bill had this incredible ability to see the bigger picture, something I struggled with. He didn't care about the imperfections I fixated on, the things I was now convinced defined me. He was just thankful to still have me by his side, no matter how much I had changed on the outside. That kind of unconditional love is indescribable. It's a small, earthly reflection of the love our Father in Heaven has for us.

With everything behind me, I could finally focus on healing—on living, recovering, and relaxing without constantly being reminded of everything I had endured. Or so I thought.

CHAPTER 19

What Would You Have Me Do?

Then a great and powerful wind tore the mountains apart and shattered the rocks before the Lord, but the Lord was not in the wind. After the wind there was an earthquake, but the Lord was not in the earthquake. After the earthquake came a fire, but the Lord was not in the fire. And after the fire came a gentle whisper.

— 1 Kings 19:11–12 NIV

A few months later, during my prayer time, I asked God what He would have me do. "What do you need me to do, Lord? Please tell me. I'll do anything. What would you have me do?"

I felt God reply with a still, small voice in my heart.

"Write a book."

Quickly, I decided that I had not heard right. I couldn't do *that*. He must have meant something else, or perhaps my own mind said that, not God. I pushed the thought away and tried to ignore it.

The trouble was, I could not ignore it. Everywhere I turned, God put more of those small coincidences in my life about writing. I began getting ads tailored for authors in my social media feed even though I had not searched for anything related to writing a book on Google. Two songs came out in rapid succession: "God is in the Details" by Big Daddy Weave and Katy Nichole and "My Story, Your Glory" by Matt West. Both songs were about God in our story, and how He can use it to reach others.

I did not want to accept what I thought God had asked me to do. So, I wrestled with it. I wrestled with God as Jacob had. Many times while praying I hear nothing, feel nothing. But when spending time on this topic, God had an answer for each of my objections.

God, I don't know what to write, I prayed.

"I will help you," came the reply.

Hardly anyone will read it, I pleaded.

"I only need one."

Because I kept feeling answers to my objections, my heart was beginning to change. I was still afraid, though. I wasn't sure I wanted to yield to what I thought God was gently nudging me toward. I did something I've never done before: I begged for a sign. *Show me you want me to write a book.* God has His ways.

My next oncology visit was only a month later. Dr. Dowell asked me about my mom, since she had treated both of us. My mom had since gone on to start radiation at a community oncology place near where my parents were staying for the remainder of the summer. I caught Dr. Dowell up on what was going on with my mom, where we were with our genetic testing and our plans, and the future of our treatment. Dr. Dowell shook her head in astonishment.

"You should write a book!"

I would have been less surprised if she had slapped me in the face. *Excuse me?* I thought, dumbfounded. I was speechless. Here was irrefutable proof, I thought, that God was listening to me and that I had heard Him correctly. How could I continue to argue with Him with this evidence? When you feel the Creator of the universe is asking you to do something, and He already died for you, how can you say no? So, I began. But I would like the record to show that I was not happy about it.

The problem was and is that I'm human. As such, I am prone to disbelief, falling away, ups and downs, exhaustion, and bad moods. All seemed to plague me. I realized that my heart was much like the Israelites in the desert.

They had witnessed miracles—plagues, the parting of the Red Sea—and still they complained. They grumbled about eating the same food day after day. They doubted. And I realized I wasn't so different. I had experienced my own share of miraculous whispers from God, and yet my confidence faltered too.

Though I had begun organizing the story in my head and had even started to consider putting words on paper, I found myself hesitating again. Doubting again. Wondering whether God had really called me to do this.

Ashamed, I asked for another sign. I felt like Gideon, the smallest and least-likely champion called by God. Gideon did not feel like a mighty hero. An angel appeared to Gideon (see Judges 6:12), and said, "The Lord is with you, mighty warrior." Gideon launched into doubt. He had some grievances about the Israelites having been pushed out of their land by another group, and then Gideon said, "My clan is the weakest in Manasseh, and I am the least in my family."

If we look at ourselves, it is easy to think, *What can I do? I'm only one person, and I am weak.*

Maybe you don't feel weak—but maybe you have another burden. Maybe you see yourself in a certain light: unable, not capable, a failure, unworthy, stuck, addicted.

But God sees beyond all that. He sees what people cannot. He sees the heart. He sees our potential.

Gideon then asked for signs from God that it was really God who was talking to him. In other, paraphrased words, "please tell me I'm not crazy, God, and give me a sign that I haven't lost my mind thinking you're talking to me." God complied. He actually gave Gideon the sign he asked for.

You would think this would give Gideon the faith to go out and fight as God had told him to do, and God had even assured Gideon that he would have victory. But it wasn't enough. Gideon had the nerve to ask God for a sign three times! Ever patient, God gave a sign each time and then (finally!) Gideon was fully on board.

Lord, help my doubting heart; I know I've already received one sign but I am not sure You've called me to write this book. Please show me that I heard You right, that You want me to do this.

Around this time my parents were selling the house that my brother and sister and I had grown up in. The house was in an idyllic location, but now two of the three siblings lived ten hours away. The house maintenance had become too much for my parents to keep up with. Their primary residence was two thousand miles away; we had only kept this house as a meeting place in the summer. My siblings and I would have liked to take the house and work on it and keep it in the family, but we had neither the capital nor the time. We all agreed, albeit begrudgingly, that it was time to sell.

Not long after that prayer, life brought a change that felt unrelated at first—but would soon become part of the answer. My parents were doing the work of going through thirty-five years' worth of life's stuff, and throwing out everything but what they absolutely could not part with. My heart went out to them for this sorting. There is a kind of mourning that comes with parting with items you are emotionally connected to. This was no easy task for them. Part of the job was going through all of their old documents.

A few weeks later, I received a letter in the mail from my mom. I was intrigued—letters weren't our usual way of communicating. We typically stuck to birthday cards, holiday greetings, and phone calls. Inside was a typed letter with a pink Post-it note attached. In her familiar handwriting, she'd written, "Came across this and wanted to send it along!" I unfolded the paper. It had been written on a word processor back in 1993, during one of her business trips to Europe.

The letter began with warm greetings, and then she offered words of encouragement—much like the angel who appeared to Gideon. Mothers have a way of knowing us deeply and accurately, sometimes better than we know ourselves. But when I reached the final line, I froze. My eyes landed on the words: "You will be a messenger for God."

I read and reread the line. I was shaken. I had asked God for another sign, and here it was, so tangible that I could literally read it. Doubt was removed. If God wanted me to do this, I would obey and step out in faith.

Which leads me to you. I have done my part by writing this book. Although I would have liked to keep these memories locked away in my heart, I am trusting God that He will reach the person He wants to reach. If any part of this helps someone, or stirs even a moment of reflection about God, it won't be because of me. That's the work of the Holy Spirit. On its own, my story isn't anything extraordinary.

Sadly, breast cancer is common. So are heart attacks. So is losing a beloved pet. What makes this story miraculous is God. Without Him, I'm just another ordinary person living an ordinary life.

Looking back, how do I feel about what I've been through? First, I believe it's made my faith stronger. We all will have crappy things happen to us. The Bible says the rain falls on the just and unjust alike (see Matthew 5:45). This means we will all experience hardships.

We will experience different trials, of course. But those trials are how and when we have the opportunity to grow the most. The two best verses when undergoing a trial are James 1:2–4, "Count it pure joy, my brothers and sisters, whenever you face trials of many kinds, because you know that the testing of your faith produces perseverance. Let perseverance finish its work so that you may be mature and complete, not lacking anything" (NIV), and Romans 5:3–5, "Not only so, but we also glory in our sufferings, because we know that suffering produces perseverance, and perseverance produces character; and character, hope. And hope does not put us to shame, because God's love has been poured out into our hearts through the Holy Spirit, who has been given to us" (NIV).

I like to focus on the good that my trials have brought. Since I am now aware of my BRCA mutation, I now get a lot more surveillance than the average person. Another benefit I see is that my children are many times more compassionate and empathetic than they have any right to be at their age. They appreciate me more. They understand that life is tenuous and that we need to celebrate being with those we love.

But even more than that, if I can bring just one person to God, I will consider it as a win. Almost a "joy." The eternal joy we are to have is described in Hebrews 12:1-3 when it says, "And let us run with perseverance the race marked out for us, fixing our eyes on Jesus, the pioneer and perfecter of faith. For the joy set before him he endured the cross, scorning its shame, and sat down at the right hand of the throne of God. Consider him who endured such opposition from sinners, so that you will not grow weary and lose heart." (NIV).

My life's race will not be the same as the next person's. It may be easier; it may be harder. I don't know what my future holds, but my specific life race is set before me for a reason and in faith, I will run my course. I will be strong and courageous—not because of anything in me, but because God makes me strong. And I know you can be, too, with God's help.

Epilogue

There is nothing special about my story. If it caused you to feel anything at all it was not by my doing but by the Holy Spirit. I know that there are millions of people who go through a cancer trial each year. Many are not as lucky as I am. If you or someone you are close to are going through your own trial right now, I am so sorry. I hope that reading this has given you some comfort to know that the God of the universe is actively watching, listening, and helping through trials both big and small. He shows up in small coincidences.

He wants to know you better, and for you to know Him better. If you would like to take a step in faith, all you need to do is recite a simple prayer asking Jesus to forgive your sins and come into your life and lead you. At the heart of it, it's that easy. I know that it seems deceptively easy. But that is why Jesus came, to make it that easy to give your heart back to Him. He's already done the hard work because God realized we'd never be able to save ourselves. Not fully.

I encourage you, if you are curious, to search for the truth. There is a lot of deception out there, and it can be hard to sift through lies, lift the veil, and determine what the truth actually is. Find a mentor, speak with a person in the clergy—anyone you can find. Lean into the questions and the doubt. God can take it. He's waiting for you. Once you find Him, He will make you strong and courageous.

Acknowledgments

I want to thank my mom for showing me what strength and courage look like, and for being my first reader.

Also, my husband and kids, who encouraged me throughout this whole journey.

I want to thank Robin at Fideli Publishing for helping with publishing and holding my hand during that entire process.

I'd like to thank Jodi Orgill Brown for her invaluable advice and for taking time she probably didn't have to read through multiple drafts. She's the strongest survivor I know.

And friends Tammy and Juanita who didn't let me back out of this venture, though I wanted to several times. God knew what he was doing when he put them in my life.

www.ingramcontent.com/pod-product-compliance
Lightning Source LLC
Chambersburg PA
CBHW071755120626
46550CB00002B/799